THE ONLY SUPPLEMENTS YOU NEED TO TRULY HELP ACHIEVE YOUR FITNESS AND HEALTH GOALS

THE LAST BOOK YOU WILL EVER BUY ON WHAT SUPPLEMENTS ARE AND WHY YOU SHOULD TAKE THEM

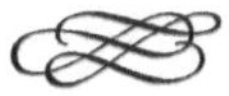

G.E.S. BOLEY JR., MBA

CONTENTS

Introduction   1

Chapter One: Supplements - The Essential Nutrients' Job   12

Chapter Two: Athletic Performance   20

Chapter Three: Vitamins   39

Chapter Four: Minerals   49

Chapter Five: Botanicals and Herbs   56

Chapter Six: Antioxidants   66

Chapter Seven: Probiotics, Weight Loss, and Feeling Great   73

Chapter Eight: Multiple Vitamin-Mineral Supplements and Essentials You Shouldn't Mix   81

Chapter Nine: Myths   88

Chapter Ten: Putting the Game Plan in Motion   97

Final Words and a Few Tasty Tidbits   105

About the Author   115

SPECIAL BONUS!   117

References   119

INTRODUCTION

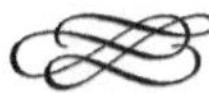

Think of all the tasks your body performs for you throughout the day …

It digests food and liquids, dispersing energy to vital systems.

It fights off bacteria and germs absorbed through the skin, lungs, and digestive tract.

It eliminates toxins and wastes, keeping your body free from decay.

It has its own cooling system to prevent overheating, which can damage vital organs.

It transmits messages from one body part to another, at a fraction of a second.

In ideal situations, all of these things are performed

moment by moment, in coordination with every cell in your body.

But what happens if cells fall short or can't complete their required task?

ALONG WITH A NUTRITIOUS DIET, OFTEN HEALTH advisors suggest supplementing nutrients with the foods you eat, so you can achieve and maintain the balance your body needs to perform at its peak. These supplementals come in a variety of consumable methods with options for customization. They are available in organic form, extracted from food sources, or synthetically reproduced by manufacturers.

By adding one or many needed supplements to your diet, you are able to attain the levels of essential nutrients your body and its systems need. By balancing your intake, you are also providing your body with balanced nutrient levels, making you feel great both inside and out.

Supplements are defined as 'essential nutrients' and are required for the body to function, grow, repair, and maintain. There are some nutrients that the body can produce with its own miraculous capabilities, but for others, it needs help in attaining the needed levels. Supplemental nutrients can be divided into 6 categories.

- Carbohydrates
- Fat
- Minerals
- Protein
- Vitamins
- Water

Carbohydrates - You've heard about carbohydrates for many years, in both good and bad scenarios. Athletes have been known to 'load up on carbs' before an athletic event, function, or game. Others have to watch their intake of carbohydrates, as they are in a weight management program and carbohydrates add unwanted stored fat (converted starch to sugars). Still again, there are other situations when health problems ask us to watch our carbohydrate intake due to cardiovascular blockage or heart disease.

The misgivings attributed to carbohydrates are extensive, and truly, some are valid, while others are exaggerated. Even when you speak with medical professionals, their opinion on carb necessities will differ. The true idea with carbohydrates is this: *the rate at which a carbohydrate raises your blood sugar determines its value in your diet.*

While it's true that carbohydrates are the body's main source of energy, sweeteners like sugar, honey, syrup, and candy, soft drinks, and cookies also contain carbohydrates, and are not the preferred 'carb' you, or your body, is in need of.

With these facts, we are reduced to reading labels on bread, pasta, and grains, such as rice or barley. We also need to pay attention to vegetables with starch in them, such as corn and potatoes, as their carbohydrates turn to sugars when digested under certain circumstances, such as the current level of energy needs or perhaps just before sleep.

Another surprise? Many fruits have carbohydrates too. And you thought you could just pick up an apple and not pay attention to its nutrition…

With fruits and whole grains, seeds, nuts, beans, and vegetables, you can also benefit from fiber content. Your body can't digest fiber, so it acts as a 'scrubber' of your digestive system. Fiber helps with constipation, and intestinal and stomach problems too.

Keep your blood sugar steady, and you have won the battle when evaluating carbohydrate intakes. Limit soda and processed foods which can contain excessive amounts of sugar. Focusing on fruits with low sugar, such as berries as well as leafy greens, will add to your nutritious diet without loading you up on calories.

Some practices to adopt to begin your awareness

• After washing, leave skins on your vegetables and fruits to retain desired nutrients

• Cereals and whole-grain breads contain fiber, make sure your choice doesn't have added sugar or molasses

• Fruit juice can have added sugars and fructose - eat whole fruits when possible

• Eat cooked lentils, beans, and peas

There are many good carbohydrates you can add to your diet program. High in fiber to help the digestive system and loaded with Vitamin Bs for absorption into the system of needed nutrients, good carbs also carry added zinc, contributing to the immunity system and cell communication. Try adding these helpful carbohydrates to add beneficial fiber to your diet

Chestnuts - lowest in fats of all nuts (less than 1 gram), chestnuts contain fiber, Vitamin C, folic acid, and are very tasty in vegetable dishes, soups, and as snacks.

Figs - 1 fig contains about 10 grams of good carbs, loaded with Vitamin Bs, calcium, potassium, and tastes great with ricotta or Greek-style yogurt.

Lentils - Low glycemic response with no sugar highs or crashes.

Oranges - Never forget oranges with their Vitamin C boost for immunity and energy, the carbs you get will taste like sunshine in the middle of winter.

Rice Bran - While most whole-grain breads are better than processed white, many have stripped the wheat of its original beneficial nutrients. Add the many gluten-sensitive people to the mix - it's your job to find a bread which is beneficial to you and can provide good carbs. Enter rice bran, with 5 grams good carbs and 2 grams fiber, it can be used in place of most whole grains to give you a truly beneficial 'whole grain' carb.

Sweet Potatoes - This is one nutrient-packed vegetable. A 4-ounce potato contains approx 143 calories, with 28 grams of carbs and more than 100% of a daily dose of beta-carotene. More than 25% of your daily intake of Vitamin C and Vitamin E will give you protection against extreme athletic environments (altitude, pollution, cold and heat) and help in recovery when you are finished. Use as you would a fresh potato, for additions to soups and chili, in 'potato' salad, and shredded raw into lean-meat meatloaf.

Fat - Fat, or lipids, are broken down into three types: saturated, monounsaturated, and polyunsaturated.

Saturated fats are mostly solid at room temperature, found in animal products and a few oils, such as coconut oil. To lower the consumption of these unwanted fats, use olive or canola oil in cooking. Replace a fatty hamburger with leaner cuts of meat and remove the skin from poultry. Eat low-fat or fat-free dairy products. Choose products with a lower saturated fat content when comparing product labels.

Monounsaturated fats have been referred to as 'the good fat' and reduce the risk of cardiovascular diseases and other health problems. They are known to usually contain the fat-soluble Vitamin E, which is also known as an antioxidant. Look to canola, olive, peanut, sunflower, and safflower oils to contain the highest amount of monounsaturated fats, as well as avocados, most nuts, and peanut butter.

Polyunsaturated fats are more nutritious than the other two fats, and often come from fish. They include omega-3 and omega-6 fats which are two of the six amino acids our bodies essentially need to function, as they promote cell growth and brain function. Besides being in fish, polyunsaturated fats can be found in cottonseed, corn, soybean and sunflower oil, seeds, and walnuts.

Although most of us don't want to have anything to do with 'fats', our bodies need them to help balance sugar levels in the bloodstream, aid our brain function (especially when stressed), build cells, help blood clotting, keep muscles supple and strong, aid in hormone regulation, and help vitamins and minerals be absorbed into the body. Fats also provide energy.

Minerals - Trace and major minerals are needed by the body, and the differentiation is the amount of each mineral needed. Major minerals are needed in larger quantities, while trace minerals are needed in smaller amounts. As you read further in this book, you will learn the benefits of these inorganic elements, as well as the many ways they help, and sometimes deter our bodies from performing at an optimum level.

These nutrients are needed by many systems within the body and can regulate basic health on a wide scale. Often, a deficiency in a mineral can lead to nerve dysfunction, unregulated blood glucose levels, or chronic diseases. There is much to learn and consider with these multi-performance system regulators.

Find essential minerals and fatty acids (often present together for related support), which can't be made by your body, in avocados, coconuts, dairy products, eggs, meats, nuts, poultry, and seafood.

Protein - Proteins are the foundation of the body. Tissues that need repair use proteins. Muscles that have been injured or fatigued need protein to regain their strength. And if you have an infection, proteins are there to fight it. Protein is also needed to supply your body with energy.

A well-balanced diet has protein built in, and supplies it through beans, eggs, seafood, lean meat and poultry. You will also find protein in soy products, nuts and seeds (unsalted). The dairy group can also supply a good portion of protein to a well-balanced diet, as well as some plant sources, which give the added benefit of containing no cholesterol, low saturated fats, and included fiber and nutrients.

There are 20 amino acids in your body, and they are all derived from protein. Hormones, antibodies and enzymes are built by protein, which is the foundation for muscle and bone strength, tones skin, supple hair, and every other part of your body which contains protein (hint- every cell in your body contains protein!).

Within the 20 amino acids, there are 9 which the body cannot produce itself, and must be supplied by the food you eat. But how much protein do we need for a balanced diet and a healthy body?

Of those remaining 11 amino acids, 6 are essential must-haves, and the body cannot function without them. These essential amino acids must either be consumed by food or with a supplement, and depend on each individual's characteristics and circumstance, which can include age, physical health conditions, pregnancy, and breastfeeding women.

Our bodies are amazing machines - consider the life of a protein. While we have been told a certain amount of protein must be consumed to achieve a balanced health standard, some proteins can be recycled from stored tissues. Other proteins are best consumed daily or as supplements, especially if a person is training for athletic fitness or specific directives by a healthcare professional. Supplements make the additional needs easy to consume and balance in the larger scheme of overall well being.

Vitamins - As you read about vitamins, you might become a bit overwhelmed by their diversity as well as their ability to affect your body's systems. While some perform well when combined with other vitamins or minerals, others do not. But fear not, there is also a section in this book which alerts you to the dos and don'ts of multivitamin and mineral combinations. Most often, unless prescribed with drugs or other essential nutrients, if taken at different times during the day, these problems can be avoided.

Vitamins are labeled in very specific ways, and as you become familiar with reading the labels, you will recognize the variances between them, minerals, and multivitamin and mineral supplements. You will also learn how vitamins have come to be identified and the many relations they have with each other and other body compounds. You will also learn about dosage amounts and how varying the supplemental intake can change another nutrients' ability to do their job.

Water - When you consider how much of our bodies are water (about 60%), it's amazing we still have to consume water each day. This is, actually, the precise reason why- to replace lost water supply through expulsion of our natural body functions, perspiration, urination, and breathing.

Our muscles and kidneys are each made of about 80% water, while our lungs tap in just over 80% and our skin at about 65%. Our brains and hearts are made of about 73% water.

All of a sudden, the need for water makes sense. To keep all of these organs and systems clean, functioning, and replacing old cells with new, it's no wonder we need clean and ample water to support these vital roles.

Water is one of the amazing overall nourishments our

bodies thrive from - it increases energy, physical performance, and mental stability. It removes wastes and toxins and keeps our skin moisturized and healthy. It is considered one of the healthiest elements we can consume.

All this without empty calories. Even more reason to love it!

While most health chronicles have a specified amount of water we each should be drinking, optimal amounts depend on a few simple guidelines, the first of which is weight.

Half your body weight, in ounces, should be consumed every day. If you weigh 160 pounds, half that is 80 pounds, converting to 80 ounces per day, needed to attain optimal functionality. By keeping this water consumption maintained, you will be guaranteeing your body is functioning at its best and chances of dehydration is minimalized. Now, you know the reasons why you carry that water bottle with you wherever you go!

You'll learn in this book how important dose size is when you are planning supplement additions to your diet. It all begins with what food you consume in your day to day diet. From there, you will construct a supplement structure to balance a diet plan to bring you to your desired end result.

When considering dose size, this book has been written with an average 19-year-old adult in mind, with no illnesses or physical deviances (the sample example used by the United States Department of Agriculture (USDA). Size of food portions and which foods to eat should be based on your own specifics, however, considering not only your age, but weight and existing conditions (pregnant, breastfeeding, chronic disease, etc.) as well as fitness goals and exercise support.

With these thoughts in mind, it is suggested by the United States Department of Agriculture (USDA) to consume the following food groups

- Dairy - 3 cups
- Fruits - 1 ½ to 2 cups
- Grains - 5 to 8 ounces
- Protein foods - 5 to 6 ½ ounces
- Oils - 5 to 7 teaspoons
- Vegetables - 2 to 3 cups

These may sound high, but if you are looking to improve your health and create a fitness program supporting an active lifestyle, you will find yourself craving these foods readily. The portions may also prove to be a bit inconvenient - while getting to know the portions and how they look on your plate, you will soon be able to eye-ball 4 ounces of grapes in no time.

Snacks - Don't forget to count that handful of almonds into your portions and the protein bar you had with that smoothie. Make sure to check the label on all processed foods (packaged items from the grocery store), breakfast items especially, as the content often has added nutrients which may throw your counts off when combining supplemental shakes or capsules. TIP: when planning and consuming snacks, put them in a bowl, don't eat them straight from the bag or sack. While you think you only have ½ cup of carrots in the bag, you may be surprised in reality, it's 1 cup and a half!

Without the addition of supplements, your body could not keep up with the demands you ask of it daily. Your body cannot produce many of its needed essential nutrients, without some kind of stimulus or intake (sunlight to produce Vitamin D, for example), so the food and supplements you consume are vital to achieving and maintaining optimal health and fitness.

Additional nutrients are especially vital if you are participating in strenuous physical and mental activities. All systems suffer when your body doesn't get the nutrients it needs - your brain functions short-circuit, your energy fails, and your immune system can become vulnerable. Your body is a fine-tuned machine and it needs a constant supply of optimum fuel to perform in the manner you request.

In this book, you will learn which supplements are needed in abundance and which ones are not. You will learn the advantages of supplements and their key role in your overall health, from boosting cell composition to improving brain performance. You will also learn how to intermingle essential nutrients for the greatest benefit when customizing your own personal diet plan.

In short, you will have all the answers to the questions you are now asking.

What minerals help strengthen my muscles?

How can I avoid joint pain or muscle cramps?

Which supplements help your body avoid illness and fatigue symptoms?

It's all here - *the last book you will ever need on supplements.*

ALWAYS REMEMBER, NO BOOK IS A SUBSTITUTE FOR professional medical advice. Please consult your healthcare provider for any serious conditions or situations you may experience. This book is provided as an informative tool only and should be used at your own discretion.

CHAPTER ONE: SUPPLEMENTS - THE ESSENTIAL NUTRIENTS' JOB

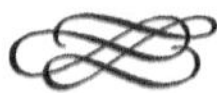

*M*y story -

"Growing up, I was never a 'strong' kid. I was skinny and felt a bit intimidated by the other boys who obviously, had more testosterone than I did. It seemed like they had more of everything.

When I turned 11, I began training in TaeKwon-Do. It didn't take long for me to find my 'home'. Finally, I'd found a place where I felt strong, agile, and in control of my own circumstances. I had a family of like-minded kids and trainers who I was taught to always respect, and in turn, respected me.

I learned not only how to move and the importance of the mind and body relationship in TaeKwon-Do, but I learned about a new world in the martial arts community as a whole. By connecting to this very special and select culture, I stepped into a world that would affect me for the rest of my life."

People are basically creatures of habit. If we've been satisfied with information from sources we are familiar with, most often we trust what will be said in the future.

Basically with some exceptions, that was the general thinking of most of us prior to the internet. Since the dawn of the 1990s, however, we have learned taking a statement at face value is to risk losing value. You may have even experienced losing your friends' respect if you quote a ridiculous fact, or losing your money to a fake internet scheme.

So, in 1994, when the Food and Drug Administration (FDA) decided to set up stipulations and guidelines for the newest trend in dietary planning, few thought it was a bad idea.

'Supplements', as they were referred to by many fitness coaches and nutritionists, became more and more important as the world realized how important the foods, specifically the nutrients and composition of our food, was. Researchers were finding by having a healthy, well-balanced diet, our bodies fended off disease and illness better, and if we exercised, ate nutrient-packed foods, and avoided bad habits, our bodies not only lived longer, but were in better condition as we aged.

For most of us, these ideas made sense, and habits were changed - a little. Some joined a fitness center while others began jogging. Aerobics became the latest activity to get into shape and see quick results, while increasing stamina and lowering blood pressure.

Along with feeling good about our fitness grew our concerns about our diet. As cancer and other disease concerns grew and we discovered how our diet affected current illness trends, knowledge about the best foods to eat and how to prepare them grew too.

The 1990s was the beginning of people awakening to not only the benefits of exercise but taking responsibility for your own diet. As we became more aware of how important exercise was, we also found the food we ate could alter our exercise effects even further. Working out for 2 hours a day so you could eat a hamburger, fries, and shake at the end of the day wasn't the most healthy of routines. We grew yet again, and craved more information to take our health to another level.

Sports and athletes became stronger. Records were being broken and even some sports regulations were considering change, as athletes accomplished what was once thought to be impossible. Had we ever imagined basketball backboards could be smashed by sheer strength alone?

As our awareness grew, the availability grew too. The produce sections at the grocer's increased and we saw vegetables and fruits we had never heard of, high in nutrients or fiber, available for purchase and consumption. We also saw increased options at the meat counter with alternative choices of grain-fed beef, free-range chicken, and steroid free meat. Fresh seafood counters were installed, with seasonal opportunities to buy multiple varieties of salmon, shrimp, and fish. You could even purchase oysters and mussels if you weren't intimidated by the preparation of such an exotic cuisine.

Some took it a step further becoming dedicated to the vegetarian or vegan lifestyle, substituting meat for other protein choices and increasing dairy and egg consumption. Many more people tried foods that had never been in their diets, such as tofu and fresh spinach.

Lifestyles were changing, and along with it, our ideas of what a 'healthy and nutritional' diet consisted of. It was no longer what was convenient, *but what was healthy.*

With each one of these new dietary choices, however, we had to learn how to prepare them.

We learned what preparation processes removed the beneficial supplements while learning how to prepare them to keep in the desired nutrients.

We learned which cooking ingredients were better for our systems – out with the shortening and in with olive oil.

We learned fried foods weighed down our digestive systems and proved to be lethal to our cardiovascular systems. Processed foods also were given a bad grade and included white sugar, processed meats with nitrates, and canned fruits using fructose corn syrup were shunned for their poor packaging processes.

Research and diet studies kept us up on the latest health advances and warnings.

Along with these changes, came supplement options. Most people had at one point or another, taken vitamins to complete their body's nutritional needs. But did we really know what was in those 'pills'?

When the guidelines for supplements were initiated, most of us just noticed all the information on the label. Few understood what riboflavin would do for our health, or what role copper played in our overall well being. Now, the consumer is much more aware of the ingredients which are contained in the foods they purchase.

You will find a 'Supplement Facts' label on every product sold as a dietary supplement, thanks to the FDA and their mandates on consumables. On this label, you will find active ingredients, the dosage amount, and additional ingredients that are listed as binders, flavorings, and perhaps fillers. Though the manufacturer of the supplement has suggested dosages, your healthcare provider may have a different dosage, considering your personal attributes. Also, be aware, the FDA does not regulate manufacturers' products and what they contain (only that they label whatever is inside). Making sure you know what you are getting in a supplement is the key to healthy choices, and is the key reason for you owning this book.

Within these pages, you are going to learn how to evaluate your regular diet by finding out what necessary nutrients are needed for optimal health. Eating nutritious meals and supplementing your diet with a balance of needed essentials will give you the advantage you need to achieve your fitness goals.

By learning what each nutrient does and how it affects your health, you will understand what supplements will benefit you most and why you should be taking them, as well as if the nutrient is better consumed in tandem or as a stand-alone dose.

You will learn the dosages which benefit you the most. You are also going to discover how these nutrients interact with your systems, other foods, and medical drugs, and why it's important to know the risks or consequences.

Companies and manufacturers of supplements must adhere to the FDA's good manufacturing practices (GMPs) which guarantee correct composition, identification, purity, and strength of dietary supplements. The GMPs are in place to prevent incorrect ingredient amounts, inappropriate label claims, and poor packaging practices.

The FDA has the right to inspect facilities that manufacture and package supplements. Remember though, the FDA does not have to approve any supplement before it can be sold, only that the claims on the label are true and any 'new dietary ingredient' (introduced after October 15 1994) provides safety evidence to the FDA before adding it to a supplement and being marketed and sold.

There are also several other agencies which monitor quality assurance, and when a manufacturer passes their standards, they are able to display seals of assurance on their packages. Though this is a good second level of approval, the seals do not guarantee the product is safe or effective. Some have even been known to produce the products they approve of, so the same runs true for supplements as other consumables you purchase - know the ingredients and choose wisely.

When you begin to understand how essential nutrients interact with your body and its systems, realizations will come to you and you will begin to understand how to plan your own fitness program. In the beginning, all the vitamins, minerals, amino acids, et all, may be a bit overwhelming. As you get to understand how these nutrients work with your body systems and what works well in combinations, you will assuredly be well on your way to planning your diet and meals with complete ease, knowing how to supplement your diet on days you may fall short or want an extra boost. Before long, you'll come to these conclusions easily and it will be second nature to you.

One of the most wonderful realizations to have with this knowledge is this - it will be with you for the rest of your life. And with it, a fit, healthy body to get you where you want to go at any stage in your life.

While reading through these chapters, you may notice many nutrients overlap from one category to another, such as Vitamin C is not only listed as a vitamin but also discussed as an antioxidant. As you familiarize yourself with the organization of this book, you will see it is divided into chapters which are segmented into the most common categories of each supplement, with additional information on how they interact and practices you may want to incorporate in your fitness plan. Descriptions also briefly name other categories each nutrient is associated with, and extends the nutrients' description according to the chapter focus.

You will also notice there is great care taken to discuss doses and how and when they should be taken with other supplements. Pay close attention to these, as some supplements cancel out other supplements' advantages, or some may heighten the effect of a particular food or drug you have ingested. All dose amounts are listed after the supplements' description, and if there is specific information about the dose, it will also be mentioned in the supplements description.

Doses stated here are based on adults, 19-year-old individuals, and if specified, will list men (M) and women (W) separately, as well as other age groups, if there is due cause. With many vitamins and some other essentials, an Upper Limit (UL) dose may be listed. This is for your fitness benefit - anything above this dose will cause detrimental risk or damage to your body and its systems.

Be aware of all supplements and nutrients, as well as drugs and medications, when designing and assembling your own program. And if you are pregnant, breastfeeding, or under the age of 18, consult your healthcare professional before beginning any supplement program.

Also, if you notice on the label any ingredient which is listed as above 200% of the daily value, research the ingredient closely. Make sure what you are consuming is safe by you and your healthcare providers' standards. Some carry little concern, but others may play a key part in your success or failure to achieve desired results.

By the time you finish this book, your knowledge for planning a healthy diet will reach into not only vitamins and minerals, but botanicals, probiotics, antioxidants, amino acids, enzymes, and multivitamins as well.

Imagine you wake up one morning feeling sluggish and achy. Because you have read this book, you'll not only know the reasons you are feeling down ... *You'll also know how to remedy the situation and get back in the game!*

CHAPTER SUMMARY

• 'Supplement' is a general term for several different essential nutrients, the most common being vitamins, minerals, botanicals/herbs, antioxidants, and probiotics.

• A supplements' effect depends largely on the composition of the ingredient and the dosage.

• Labels of supplements must contain specific information, as these ingredients aren't regulated by the FDA, just their inclusion. Label information helps the consumer determine the appropriateness and purity of its contents.

IN THE NEXT CHAPTER, LABELING AND DEFINITIONS WILL be discussed in depth, giving you the needed information to make wise choices when considering supplements for your fitness program.

CHAPTER TWO: ATHLETIC PERFORMANCE

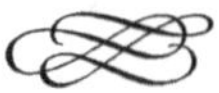

"While training for a spot on the ITF TaeKwon-Do US Team and eventually competing at the World Championship held in Seoul Korea in 2003, I dedicated myself to doing everything I could possibly do to become the most fit, the most powerful, and the most keenly attuned athlete I could become.

I'd been diligently training for over two years, and as I drove to the competition tryouts in Connecticut, I felt confident in my well-organized plan. I had even packed all my specific foods and supplements I'd been consuming so I wouldn't throw any of my systems off or lose any ground if the same diet couldn't be found.

If I had to substitute one of my favored foods or essentials for something of lesser worth, I knew my performance would suffer. I was sure by continuing the same diet and regimen I had been using while training, my mind, body, and soul would be ready for anything I was faced with.

I couldn't have been more wrong ... "

When you are an athlete, or just want to be in shape like one, *performance* is your main focus. You want top performance from your body, beginning with the strength of your muscles, the flexibility of your joints to the clarity of your thoughts. But because 'athletic performance' addresses the fitness group as a whole, what may be a great supplement for a runner won't exactly be a great supplement for a wrestler.

More and more, however, products are being formulated for specific sports and activities. If there's anything the manufacturers know, it's how to appeal to a sensitive, intelligent community, and athletes are at the top of the list. Even yogis have a specific focus for their diet, and supplements play a role in balancing their diet planning too.

While we are talking about manufacturers, it may interest you to know, most of them do not run trials or studies which prove combination success or singular advantage. They often formulate their products with the current 'trend' or sell to specific regions due to their current marketing, instead of producing products that will benefit the consumer.

This lack of awareness just means as a purchaser, you must be educated on what you need in your diet as well as the combinations' benefit or disadvantage of consuming the dosage at the same time. The popularity of a trend gains marketing attention over a responsive combination of supplemental nutrients. Be prudent and diligent in your attention.

Let's put this idea into a real-life situation. Picture a medium-sized town, where the college supports about 25% of the jobs. Our college is large enough to have fall sports - men's soccer and football. Winter sports, such as men's and women's basketball. Spring sports which include track and field and women's soccer, and summer softball and baseball. During each of these seasonal sports, they have particular product packages directed at specific markets, though the contents of the package are exactly the same product. Fall promotes muscle strength, winter promotes high energy and stamina, spring promotes strength and endurance, and summer promotes keen muscle reaction and brain function.

While the manufacturing of the supplement remains the same, the label changes due to market demand and preference.

It's not to say consumers don't like this … we do. And because supplements have expiration dates, manufacturers are easily set up to appeal to their target audience, with a selling advantage over a generally packaged or single nutrient labeled product that loses its potency while waiting to be purchased.

In addition to this sleight of hand for consumers, they also tend to exaggerate the results with terms like 'be in the best health possible' or 'run faster than you ever have before'. And true, these statements could be the truth, but generally, they are ploys and should be understood as such. If there is anything you have learned up to this point, it's the benefits, advantages, and mastery of essential nutrients and how they affect your body's systems. Don't succumb to the shallow claims of a marketing campaign.

Use this knowledge when reading athletic and high-performance supplement labels.

An idea to also note is this. Many supplemental companies come and go throughout a one- or two-year product life span. In other words, they will start a company and market a brand for as long as it sells well. When the brand begins to decline, the manufacturer changes their label and launches a 'new' product, which is basically the same product with the latest trend statements and benefits promoted.

If the brand or manufacturer of a supplement you are looking to begin has been around for a while, you can be fairly sure it is a reputable and long-lasting producer, providing the claimed advantages to its consumer audience. If, however, the manufacturer is a new, explosive, and 'quick sell' marketer, be aware of the ingredients and their shelf life.

Supplements can be expensive, make sure you are putting your money when it will do you the most good.

Remember, the FDA regulates these performance supplements just as it does vitamins and minerals. In other words, there is no testing or approval of performance claims of these supplements. It is left to the manufacturer to provide safe supplement information content and ensure the statements on the label are truthful. If it is found claims are misleading or not manufactured in the ways stated, the FDA as well as the Federal Trade Commission (FTC) can take action against these businesses and producers which make false claims about performance and results.

It is of great importance to also know, when buying products online or internationally, to be aware of products manufactured in other countries. Quite often they are empty products with little or no nutritional worth, yet claim to have incredible results. There are no standards of packaging or manufacturing of the products, and have also been known to contain harmful substances. It's bad enough they don't give you what they claim, but to get ingredients that can break down your bodies' systems is a painful and sometimes, irreversible lesson to learn.

A word about steroids -

A new trend among supplements aimed at high-performance consumers is 'legal steroids' and claim they do not show up in drug tests and are legal to use. The labels have also been found to list ingredients that allude to the idea they are anabolic steroids. As in some cases for drug testing, anabolic steroids are illegal. Is there a way to detect the difference?

The United States Drug Enforcement Administration (DEA) has listed many anabolic steroids - compounds that are designed to act as testosterone does. Some of these supplemental products are categorized as controlled substances and are regulated by the DEA. If you are suspicious of any ingredient, check out the DEA's list of controlled substances. But even then, be careful you are not consuming a chemical that will violate state and federal laws. Or worse, damage your body in ways which can't be repaired.

As we explore the wide range of supplements aimed at body performance, keep in mind your own desires and what you think will benefit or deter you from your focus. Most products directed at athletes and performance achievers will be a combination of supplements, very much like multivitamin and minerals (MVM's) supplements, and are available as powders, capsules, liquids, gel tabs, and tablets. Some require you to take them throughout the day, others are a one-shot dosage to last the duration. Others still may even be a monthly dosage, which is likely to contain fat-soluble vitamins and slow-release minerals which you don't want to overindulge with. Good judgment will benefit you in your choices for your desired results.

It is a good adage to know, though performance supplements are available in many forms, by consuming these supplements in liquid or gel form (powders also considered liquid once mixed), you'll be getting the nutrients in your bloodstream and to the end result quicker, thereby utilizing their advantages quicker, than if taken by tablet form. Because these products aren't regulated, some have even been known to be excreted without much breakdown at all, as can be the case with pills and tablets. The price of these products is too high to put your trust into the unknown.

You will notice some of these essential nutrients are covered in other chapters in the book with more descriptions, under their designed category, and have a more thorough description, They are found in their specific category, such as vitamins or botanicals. The discussion here will be focused on the sense of performance, rather than the body's overall benefits of the supplement. Individual compounds specific to performance supplements only will be described thoroughly, with advantages and disadvantages listed as well.

The recommended dosage for adults is listed with each description for a 19-year-old, M for average adult men and W for average adult women. If no gender is listed, it benefits both sexes the same. The upper limit dosage (UL) is often the high-performance level and will be what is listed here. It is suggested you do not exceed the dosage amounts. These doses are measured in milligrams (mg), micrograms (mcg), grams (g) or international units (IU), depending on the nutrient, and are *daily intake levels*, unless otherwise mentioned.

Antioxidants - (Referring to Vitamin C, Vitamin E, and coenzyme Q10 specifically) If you participate in sports regularly, it is a good chance you breathe more heavily and to a deeper capacity than a person who doesn't participate in athletics regularly. Because of this intense and deep breathing, it is thought you take in more free radicals than an average person, putting your muscles and cells at risk. By consuming antioxidants, and there are many to choose from, you can counter this occurrence, and thereby reduce inflammation, muscle aches, and fatigue. Please refer to each specific nutrient (such as green tea or Vit C) for the upper level (UL) dosage for performance and advantages, but be aware of any combination warnings between these essential nutrients.

Arginine - Like other amino acids, arginine is found in foods that contain protein - dairy products, eggs, fish, meat, and poultry. Studies have shown little to no benefit of this nutrient, though many athletes swear by its claims, which are noted for strength building (bodybuilding), improved performance, and aerobic benefits (running and cycling). Suggested dosages for both men and women are 2 to 20 g for 3 months.

Beetroot or beet juice - Due to it being one of the best sources for nitrate, beetroot or beet juice can improve athletic performance. Nitric oxide expands blood vessels, thereby increasing blood circulation and flow to the muscles. Increased blood flow also improves the removal of waste products which cause muscle fatigue. Usually focused on runners, aerobic sports, and recreational athletes. This antioxidant may turn your urine pink or red. 2 cups of juice 2 to 3 hours before exercise. No cautions.

Beta-alanine - This amino acid is found in fish, meat, and poultry. Most diets have about 1 gram a day of beta-alanine which is used to make carnosine for skeletal muscles in your body. Extended exercise produces lactic acid, reducing muscular strength and can cause fatigue and loss of energy. Carnosine can reduce the buildup of lactic acid, The amount of carnosine produced by each person from beta-alanine is individual and varies from person to person. It has been tested in swimmers and team sports which focus on muscle fatigue and strength required for high-intensity and intermittent efforts over short periods of time. Results are inconclusive. Doses of 800 mg have been found to produce severe paresthesia, a tingling, prickling, or burning sensation in the face, neck, upper torso, and back of the hands, lasting 60 to 90 minutes. The effect has not been considered harmful and passes with elimination.

Beta-hydroxy-beta-methylbutyrate (HMB) - The amino acid leucine, found in foods and protein powders, is converted in the body to HMB. Conversion by the liver further transforms the HMB into another compound thought to help muscle cells restore structure and function after exertion. Recovery in athletes is of particular interest and is where the most benefit has shown results, especially if exertion is intense and over a long period of time, such as in marathon runners or sport cyclists. 3 g per day up to 8 weeks; also available with calcium (400 mg).

Betaine - If you are consuming a nutritious diet of normal activity, you are probably consuming 100 to 300 mg a day of betaine. Though it hasn't been proven to affect or improve athletic performance, many bodybuilders and athletes looking for power performance often add betaine to their supplements regime. No side-effects have been found. 2 g to 5 g per day, up to 15 days.

Branched-chain amino acids (BCAAs) - The amino acids referred to as BCAA's include leucine, isoleucine, and valine, and are found in a nutritious diet containing animal foods, such as meat and milk. Muscles use these amino acids during exertion for support and to replenish cells. It is thought by adding this supplement while performing endurance sports, such as distance running and marathon sports, it will improve strength and muscle tone. Though a nutritious diet usually contains enough BCAA's to support balance, if you are looking for performance achievement, a supplement of the BCAA's will likely be of benefit. 20 g per day as a supplement.

Caffeine - As caffeine is a stimulant, it is often paired with other high-performance nutrients to intensify the benefit, if only for a minimal time period. There may be more than one reason you body craves that cup of coffee in the morning - coffee has high levels of antioxidants that contribute to brain health as well as increasing neurotransmitters like serotonin. Your mood is enhanced by caffeine's ability to block adenosine, a chemical agent that causes drowsiness. Coffee, with its natural caffeine, is also known to sharpen concentration and is linked to reducing the risk of many neurological diseases. Endurance and fatigue reduction are its sought after benefits, found naturally in coffee, tea, guarana and kola nuts, but also found in high amounts in energy drinks and supplements. It has not shown to be of any benefit in short, intense exercise, however, and doesn't boost performance in everyone. Athletic experts agree caffeine helps to maintain intense levels of exercise and reduces feelings of fatigue. consuming higher doses than the upper limit could prove to be detrimental and more often reduces physical performance rather than improves it, while also disturbing sleep routines. It can also cause irritability and anxiety if consumption is of a higher dosage. 2 to 6 mg per kilogram of body weight 15 to 60 minutes before exercise can increase training time. 400 to 500 mg per day, teenagers should not exceed 100 mg per day. UL 500 mg *10,000 mg in a single dose (1 tablespoon of pure caffeine powder) can be fatal.* NOTE: The National Collegiate Athletic Association and International Olympic Committee limit amounts of caffeine ingested before competitions.

Citrulline - This is another amino acid your body produces and is also found in many common foods. Kidneys convert citrulline into other amino acids, namely arginine, which transforms into nitric oxide and expands your blood vessels. Blood flow is increased, delivering oxygen and nutrients to muscles. This improves strength and energy while also removing wastes. Research results are limited - some users have experienced stomach discomfort while taking it. 9 g as a single dose, or 6 g per day for 16 days.

Creatine - A compound that is stored in your muscles, creatine supplies energy, and in supplemental doses, can improve performance. Creatine monohydrate, perhaps the most widely studied and used form of creatine in supplements, can be found in natural foods like beef and salmon, but the body also produces about 1 gram daily by itself. Supplements of creatine have been known to increase strength, power, and the ability to contract muscles for maximum effort. When taken over several weeks or months, it can help with training, enhancing performance during repeated short bursts of intense intermittent activity and lasts up to close to 3 minutes at a time, as needed when weight lifting or sprinting. Due to its water-retentive tendencies, it is often associated with a bit of weight gain, but over the long term, has shown little to no detrimental side-effects, though there have been rare cases of muscle stiffness and cramps, as well as GI distress. Loading dose of 20 g per day (4 equal doses throughout) for 5 to 7 days, and then maintenance of 3 to 5 g per day.

Dehydroepiandrosterone (DHEA) - As a steroid hormone produced by the adrenal glands, DHEA is a male hormone that increases muscle strength and size. DHEA has not been found to improve any strength or aerobic capacity, nor does it raise testosterone levels, as it often is labeled as doing. The National Collegiate Athletic Association and the World Anti-Doping Agency prohibits the use of DHEA in athletic competitions. DHEA is not prohibited by military service members, except the Coast Guard. When taken by females, DHEA increases testosterone and in turn, can cause facial hair growth and acne. Also labeled as Prasterone (synthetic) and Androstenolone, it is often bundled together with other supplements when 'stacking', a practice which can cause major body discomfort, irritability, and intense agitated mood swings. Stacking is highly discouraged for any physical exercise.

Ginseng - Though most don't know, there are a few types of ginseng - Panax, also known as American, Chinese, Japanese, or Korean ginseng, has been thought to improve stamina and vitality. Russian, or Siberian ginseng, has been used to strengthen the immune system and ward off fatigue. When considering athletic performance and athletic exercise, neither ginseng has been found to be of any benefit, though both are deemed safe to use. In supplemental form, headaches and sleep disruptions have been known to occur, but no other side-effects have been recorded.

Glutamine - Yet another amino acid your body uses to produce energy. It is promoted as a performance enhancer and strengthens muscle-building and recovery, though little scientific proof is available to support this claim. Body-builders are the most popular group of athletes to take this supplement. It is found as an essential nutrient in protein powders and tablets, and many athletes believe its claims.

Iron - As a mineral, iron has been found to deliver oxygen to muscles and tissues and it is wanted for the same benefits as a performance enhancer. By oxygenating tissues, cells use the iron to assimilate food into energy and eliminate iron deficiencies. This is of high concern, especially if an athlete is feeling tired and has reduced performance. Because of the lengthy process of iron increase to optimum levels, if an athlete is depleted, activity may have to stop in order for the body to assimilate the iron and recover to needed levels. If more than 45 mg of iron is consumed per day, digestive tracts can be compromised. Doses in supplements to treat anemia can improve exercise capacity, but a healthcare provider should be monitoring levels to assure its success. 13 to 19 years of age - M 11 mg, 13 to 19 W 15 mg; 20 - 50 M 8 mg, 20 - 50 W 18 mg; 51+ M and W 8 mg; UL 40 mg

Ketones - Naturally, this molecule is made in the liver and comes from the stored fat when the body doesn't receive nourishment for a long period of time, about 72 hours. Exogenous ketones, or synthetic ketone supplements, are labeled as enhancing physical performance, mental perfor-mance, and weight loss, and vary with dose, depending on the results you want. They have become quite popular with athletes who follow a strict ketogenic diet when restricting carbohydrate intake to produce higher levels of ketones. They usually contain beta-hydroxybutyrate (BHB), medium-chain triglycerides (MCT) or both. When added with minerals, you will see them labeled as 'ketone salts' or with other supplements in liquid form as 'ketone esters'. While there is little to no scientific evidence supporting the effectiveness of ketone supplements, side effects have been limited to the digestive tract - diarrhea, indigestion, and vomiting.

Nootropics - These are known as substances intended to improve mental performance, and are also known as 'brain boosters', 'cognitive enhancers', 'memory enhancers', and 'smart drugs'. To be called a nootropic, the chemical (always synthetic) has to enhance memory, help brain function, protect the brain, and is relatively safe. Some nutrients can help in several of these areas, but there is no known substance that can help in all areas. Thus, nootropics are highly suspicious in the supplement arena, until more studies and research proves otherwise. Added ingredients to a nootropics' label may include harmful ingredients or drugs, and it is strongly suggested to research all ingredients and their tendencies before making them a part of your fitness diet plan.

Protein - Though we've talked about protein and its role as a supplement, many athletes and sports enthusiasts proclaim its benefits are mainly in performance-related roles, but it has many other benefits too. As protein builds, maintains, and repairs muscle tissue, because of its cell strengthening qualities, it is also loved for the enhanced recovery benefits, thereby shortening muscle healing and recovery between athletic exertion. Essential amino acids (EAAs) which are in proteins, can be found in many foods, and some amino acids can only be made by the body which come only from foods. Some of the highest concentrations of nutrients and vitamins are found in whole eggs, and help brains to function at peak performance. They contain a beneficial compound called choline, a micronutrient that creates acetyl-choline (the neurotransmitter regulating mood and memory) which is packed in the yolk. Dairy products, eggs, fish, meat, and poultry provide needed amino acids, but some can only be found in plant foods - grains and legumes are good examples. Most protein supplements contain whey, a protein which is found in milk, and amazingly, provides all the EAAs a normal body needs. Athletes need from 0.5 to 0.9 g of protein per pound of body weight per day (a 150-pound person would need 75 g to 135 g per day). During heavy or intense training, more may be needed in order to maintain your health and muscle mass. High consumption of protein doesn't have any side effects, though there is no benefit to it either (some trainers suggest protein doses up to .14 g per pound of body weight from multiple sources every 2 to 3 hours per day).

Quercetin - This is a compound found in some beverages (tea, for example), fruits, and vegetables. Quercetin is suggested to increase energy production in muscles and improves the circulatory system, though studies and research has been inclusive. Benefits are minimal. 1000 mg per day for 8 weeks

Ribose - Ribose helps muscles produce more energy and is a natural sugar in your body. Research studies are few, so to come to any conclusive information is premature. The studies which have been conducted showed little benefit from doses ranging from 625 mg to 10,000 mg per day up to 8 weeks. Because so few have studied ribose, a safe or beneficial dose is unknown, but no side effects have yet to be documented.

Sodium bicarbonate (baking soda) - Sodium bicarbonate reduces the buildup of acids, which accumulate after intense exercise over several minutes. The reduced muscle force and tiredness from strenuous activities is a recurring condition in sprinters and swimmers, so sodium bicarbonate has proven to be a relieving source for them. Intermittently intense sports, such as Mixed Martial Arts (MMA), kickboxing, boxing and tennis, have also appreciated its benefits. Some athletes have developed different responses, which can hinder or reduce performance. GI distress (nausea and vomiting) has been caused by sodium bicarbonate in some athletes, along with weight gain (due to water retention). 300 mg per kilogram of body weight is suggested, or 4 to 5 teaspoons of baking soda per day.

Tart or sour cherry - The Montmorency Cherry variety has compounds in them which may ease recovery from extreme exercise. They can reduce pain and muscle damage from strength-related activities, and can ease lung trauma from endurance activities, such as marathon or triathlon events, which require heavy breathing. Bodybuilders have been known to recover their strength with little or no muscle soreness or fatigue with this supplement, though once again, studies have been few. It is also thought tart cherry may help runners race faster and experience fewer lung compromises after a marathon or event. 2 cups of juice (or 500 mg of tart cherry skin powder) for 1 week before the exercise and continue consumption for 2 days after to aid recovery.

Tribulus Terrestris - This is a plant whose compounds are labeled to improve performance by increasing levels of many hormones, including testosterone. Research is limited, though in studies, high doses have caused heart, kidney, and liver damage in animals. Tribulus terrestris is found as an added nutrient in performance powders and tablets.

Whey Protein - When considering whey comes from cows milk, it is easily consumed in natural foods Whey products, such as powdered supplements or additives, are sold in gels, ready-to-drink shakes, sport and energy bars, and other food products. It is often taken to support an already protein-rich diet when muscle growth and repair is desired. All the essential amino acids (EAA) are found in milk, but if you have an allergy to cow or dairy products, this would be a good supplement to incorporate. It is considered to be a higher form of protein supplement than its cousins, casein and soy, because it is digested faster, leading to quicker absorption of the needed amino acids. Be aware most whey supplements have added ingredients, which may conflict with other aspects of your essential nutrients and diet. NOTE - It will be a futile task to take whey supplements to exceed your already rich protein diet. There are no benefits for additional whey products when wanting to boost performance, but if you find you are lacking in the essential proteins it offers, it is a good way to balance your needed levels.

Any supplement can have side effects and could interact with other prescriptions, remedies, and over-the-counter medications. As we've mentioned before, know your ingredients, especially when taking compound or multi-nutrient supplements. Athletes are known to be in tune with their bodies - pay close attention to the dose and effects all supplements may have on your performance and day to day living. By adding or eliminating a supplement individually, it is easier to see its effect on your body, its systems, and your performance.

Some side effects which are signs your body is giving you that something is amiss, are nausea, vomiting, shakiness, rapid or irregular heart rate, chest pain, headaches, shortness of breath, mood or changes in behavior, and yellowing of the skin or eyes (indicating liver trouble). If you have any of these conditions or have questions, always consult a health-care professional.

Be especially aware of the supplements you take if you are competing, and also if those supplements are in multi- or compound doses. The FDA prohibits certain ingredients some performance dietary supplements used to contain, such as androstenedione, dimethylamylamine (DMA), and ephedra. Other products may contain unlawful stimulants, hormone-like ingredients, prescription medications, unapproved drugs, or steroids. Not only will these substances disqualify you from competition, but they are dangerous and can cause health issues while taking them and for many years after.

Scams - As we mentioned briefly before, yes, they are out there, and more prolific than you would ever suspect - the Performance Supplements and Bodybuilding industries are main targets for these criminals. Many false claims are being stated on labels and products, and the FDA can't be everywhere at all times, especially when the products are sold online and are produced in foreign countries.

These scammers are also becoming more sophisticated and tech-savvy, making it that much harder to identify them to trusting consumers. Here are a few notorious scams which have not only dupped innocent purchasers out of their money, but they've also left many people with detrimental health conditions, including permanent damage to the liver and heart.

False Representatives from the FDA - These people have gathered your information from a list of purchasers who have ordered pharmaceuticals and supplements online, from catalogs, or over the phone. The person calling will claim you have purchased illegal contraband and, unless you pay the associated fee, you will be subject to a subpoena, house searches, or arrest. They are also very savvy about having local or national phone numbers which you may recognize on your phone screen thinking their claims are true, though in all actuality, they are located outside the USA (most recently in the Dominican Republic). No representatives will call from the FDA, and as with all agencies, will not ask for money from you. If you suspect fraud, hang up. The website of the FDA has more information concerning these calls and fraudulent activity.

Claims on Product Labels and Promotions - We've all seen the late-night infomercials claiming miracle products to cure disease or weight loss programs, promising weight loss of 30 lbs. in 30 days or hair regrowth within 14 days.

But what happens if you do fall victim to these claims and find out afterward you've been scammed?

Most often, you will only be out the price. But more and more people are seeing health issues associated with these products, especially with a system referred to as 'stacking', where the manufacturer sells you multiple products to give you quicker results. Not only are manufacturers putting inert ingredients in, such as sugar or sodium, but they are also adding unknown ingredients which may, on a short term basis, give you a stimulating feeling or ease your ailments. But they are short-lived, leading to other conditions.

Side effects from fraudulent manufacturers have included irritability, digestive upset, and headaches, but more risky conditions have also been documented, such as liver damage and increased heart disease. The best solution is to make sure you purchase any medications from a licensed pharmacist, and if you are taking medical prescriptions, to only take supplements endorsed by your trainer or medical profes-sional. Anything less, and you are literally, putting your health into an unknown person's hands.

With all the potential places we can see scams, it's good practice to become aware of some basic tactics of a predatory fraud. Here are some key points to be aware of if you shop online or by phone, and suspect a scam or fraudulent product.

False or Bold Claims - Most often, there will be false

claims made, such as 'cure' for diabetes or 'improves sexual performance overnight'.

Personal Testimonials - These will range from 'Cured my Arthritis!' to 'I don't have Diabetes Anymore!' ... anything which sounds this good is probably, as you well know, too good to be true.

Uses Scientific Wording - These statements will often use 'breakthrough' 'new research has been discovered', 'secret formula', or 'all-natural cure'. They are playing on hopes of people who want new answers and revised hope. Don't fall for them.

Use your head, not your heart when you purchase supplements, and always, follow your trainer's suggestions. They have the newest and best information when it comes to your supplements and won't fill you with false ideas or unattainable goals.

Performing at your peak and recovering quickly is important to any athlete, whether recreational or competitive. The wise athlete will eat a nutritionally balanced diet, supplement to meet balances, drink enough fluids to stay hydrated, assure physical fitness, and have a well- planned fitness program. Scientific evidence for performance supplements are still in their infancy, and to judge any by word of mouth or label statements without verifying with a professional trainer or medical professional is a potential case for harm. Obtain guidance from a sports-medicine expert or trainer if you have specific questions about your own diet plan or exercise routine.

Don't compromise your health and performance with misinformation and assumed strategies. Being fit is the best thing you can do for your wellbeing and positive outlook. Keep the supplements nutritious, and you'll experience the highest level of fitness you've ever known!

Chapter Summary

• Because the FDA doesn't regulate supplements, making sure you know what you are getting is the key to healthy and beneficial choices.

• Nutrients and ingredients must be listed on every supplemental label, as well as nutritional value and required statements.

• Adding supplements to your health plan will give your body the balance in essential nutrients it needs to perform at optimum levels.

IN THE NEXT CHAPTER, YOU WILL LEARN WHAT VITAMINS are, how they affect your system, and the pros and cons of the most common vitamins used.

CHAPTER THREE: VITAMINS

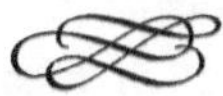

"*After a disastrous showing at the 2003 ITF TaeKwon-Do United States Nationals, I was determined to find out why I had a bad showing. Why did I feel exhausted when I hadn't while I was training? Why was my anxiety level high? I felt confident in my training and with my performance before the actual competitions. And why couldn't I regain my composure and level of performance when I tried to restructure my strategy?*

All of this could be answered, and was, with one simple change. After I had researched how the body performs when under stress and with increased levels of fatigue, the light came on and I restructured my game plan from that day forward. It made all the difference in the world."

Vitamins play an important part in our body's overall health. They affect almost every part of our body in one way or another – from strengthening bones to improving eyesight. They are probably the most popular supplements people take, and most of us know the basic advantages of the common vitamins, like Vitamin D is good for your bones and Vitamin A is good for eyesight.

Vitamins are categorized into two groups, *water-soluble,* meaning your body doesn't store them and they are excreted if not needed. These vitamins usually need replenishment every two to three days, though some like Vitamin C and B12 can be temporarily stored for longer periods of time. They also help free up the nutrients of the food you've eaten, while also keeping tissues healthy.

Fat-soluble vitamins, which mean they are stored in your body's' fat, and are used when needed, and move through your system on proteins, such as lymph channels in the intestinal wall to gain access to the bloodstream. Oils and fatty foods can be reservoirs for several of these vitamins, as well as being stored in the fat tissues of the liver for later needs. Minimal consumption of these vitamins is usually the plan as your body gradually dispenses them as your body's needs arise. Use these vitamins minimally, as toxic levels can build up in body storehouses if you over-consume, easily done with unmonitored supplements.

Make sure, if you are eating breakfast cereals or bars, quite often they have added vitamins and minerals to their natural nutrition. Breakfast beverages, or fitness drinks may also have added ingredients affecting your supplemental tally. There are some vitamins which more is not necessarily better, so make note of your food intake and check the labels before putting a supplemental plan in place - you may be getting more supplements than you are aware of.

Labeling of vitamins uses letters from the alphabet, such as vitamins A, B, C, and so on. Some vitamins, such as B and D, have numbers as well, indicating they have the same basic molecular composition, but still differ slightly. As the medical world evolved, so did the discovery of compounds and supplements used to treat illnesses, and as these practices improved and more knowledge was gained, many labeled vitamins were re-categorized under their more appropriate place. Let's discuss the ones you will find most beneficial to your fitness and health.

The recommended dosage for adults is listed with each description for a 19-year-old, M for average adult men and W for average adult women. The upper limit dosage (UL) recommended, will be listed last. If you find there is no 'upper limit' listed, then it is undetermined at this time. These dosages are the Institute of Medicine's Recommended Daily Amount (RDA), in milligrams (mg), micrograms (mcg), or international units (IU), depending on the nutrient.

Vitamin A – One of the first molecule compounds (vitamins) to be discovered, Vitamin A is a fat-soluble retinoid (preformed), metabolized by the body, and includes retinol, retinal, and retinyl esters. Among the benefits of Vitamin A are support for the immune system, eyesight and vision, communication between cells, and the reproductive system. *Preformed Vitamin A* can be found in foods from animals, such as dairy products, meat (higher levels in the liver) and fish.

Provitamin A (carotenoids) mostly found in vegetables and leafy greens, is converted in the body if there are low levels of Vitamin A. Determining levels of intake can be tricky, It is important to pay close attention to what you eat. A supplemental regimen of Vitamin A can help support the systems in your body to maintain optimum health, but unused Vitamin A, which is stored in the liver, can accumulate, causing liver damage if not regulated.

Vitamin A, in multivitamins as well as a standalone supplement, is often labeled as retinyl acetate or retinyl palmitate, or in some forms as beta-carotene. The amounts of Vitamin A vary and are often found in higher doses in children's and senior's multivitamins as their livers do not function at optimum levels, as do adults. M 900 mcg, W 700 mcg, UL 3000 mcg.

Vitamin B – A deficiency of Vitamin B is perhaps the most obvious of all the supplements reactions, due to its role at maintaining cell health. Low energy, fatigue, and confusion are most noticeable, but anemia or compromised immune systems can also be a result from low Vitamin B intake.

Due to the many types of Vitamin B available, each has a specific effect on different systems within the body. And because the family of Vitamin B has so many compound differences, many were named as one supplement, only to be discovered as medicine evolved, it was a Vitamin B relative. Some of the derivative names may be familiar to you!

Vitamin B1 (Thiamin) – Vitamin B1 converts food into energy and is beneficial to the nervous system. Vitamin B1 is a water-soluble vitamin and can be found in whole grains, dark green vegetables, eggs, and milk. Consuming alcohol can prevent the absorption of Vitamin B1, which is why you may have heard taking Vitamin B1 helps to reduce the symptoms of over-indulging alcohol. It doesn't actually, but having the extra Vitamin B1 in your system could help sustain needed levels if it outlasts the alcohol in the system. M 1.2 mg, W 1.1 mg

Vitamin B2 (Riboflavin) – This water-soluble vitamin also converts food to energy while also helping to maintain proper eyesight. If a person abuses alcohol, however, Vitamin B2 is hard to absorb and can show up as a deficiency with dryness around the corners of the mouth. M 1.3 mg W 1.1 mg

Vitamin B3 (Niacin) – Once again, this water-soluble vitamin helps convert food into energy and also aids in promoting a healthy appetite and proper digestion. Vitamin B3 can be found in chicken, liver, red meat, fish, peanuts, wheat, and barley. If you don't consume enough Vitamin B3 in your diet, a supplement is of great benefit. You will avoid nausea and abdominal cramps, and in extreme cases, confusion, by adding this digestive benefactor to your diet plan. M 16 mg, W 14 mg, UL 35 mg

Note: a derivative of Niacin, Nicotinamide riboside (NR) and Nicotinamide mononucleotide (NMN) which are produced in the body, have been known to play a critical part in energy metabolism, DNA repair, and gene expression, giving them the values of cell restructure and system function. Oral consumption of these supplements have shown improved energy levels, decrease of age-associated genetic changes, and possibly insulin sensitivity. More research, however, needs to be done before these statements are decisive.

Vitamin B5 (Pantothenic acid) – This vitamin also converts food into energy and aids in creating lipids (fats). It also is a key component of increasing neurotransmitters (brain function and neuron communication), steroid hormones (contributing to strength and agility), and hemoglobin (blood health and clotting properties). Vitamin B5 also slows mental decline as well as aiding in suppressing depression in aging adults. It synthesizes brain chemicals too, and regulates sugar levels. While found in many common diet foods, such as chicken, eggs, and tomatoes, you'll often see this water-soluble vitamin listed on multivitamin labels, as the trace elements of Vitamin B5 are easier to list than to try and remove. M 5 mg, W 5 mg

Vitamin B6 (Pyridoxine) – This water-soluble vitamin aids in converting food into energy, but also helps in fighting off infection in the body. If you are pregnant or breastfeeding, by having a balanced dose of B6 in your diet, you will also be helping your baby's brain development. Not only will you find B6 in whole grains and red meats, but tuna and salmon contain Vitamin B6 as well as several fruits and vegetables, including watermelon, chickpeas, spinach, and potatoes. Be wary of excess intake of B6, as very high doses can cause nerve damage, numbness, and muscle weakness. 30 to 50 years old, M 1.3 mg, W 1.3 mg; 50+, M 1.7 mg, W 1.5; UL 100 mg

Vitamin B7 (Biotin or Coenzyme R) – Please see Vitamin H, below.

Vitamin B9 (Folic acid or Folate) – Vitamin B9, a water-soluble vitamin, helps the growth of red blood cells and reduces the risk of birth defects, specifically in the spine and brain, when consumed during pregnancy. Folic acid is the synthetic form found in processed foods, such as cereals, whereas Folate is found naturally – meats, organ meats, legumes, fish, beets, and leafy green vegetables. If you don't consume these foods and digest enough folate, the lack can be recognized by diarrhea or anemia. Supplements are easily attained and will tend to your deficiency easily. M 400 mcg, W 400 mcg, UL 1000 mcg

Vitamin B12 (Cobalamin) Not only does B12 contribute substantially to forming red blood cells and DNA, but it also helps to regulate your nervous system. It is water-soluble and is absorbed in the intestines. If you are a vegetarian, it is easy to drop below the needed levels of B12, as the most naturally consumed B12 foods are red meat, organ meat, fish and shellfish, but also include cheese, and eggs. If you are running low on this vitamin, supplementals are highly recommended. A lack of B12 will show in the nervous system, such as dementia, paranoia. confusion and depression, especially in senior-aged adults. Other symptoms of low B12 include a pins-and-needles effect in the hands and feet, irritability or depression, extreme fatigue, and weakness or exhaustion. Because Vitamin B12 plays such an integral role in vital systems of your body, it is advised if any of the above conditions occur, see a physician to determine the cause. M 2.4 mcg, W 2.4 mcg

Vitamin C – There are many advantages to having healthy levels of Vitamin C in your system. It is a strong antioxidant that helps your natural defenses against chronic diseases, such as heart disease. It also protects cells and boosts your immune system, and by increasing antioxidant blood levels, it helps your body fight inflammation. Vitamin C found in oranges is also a key factor in preventing mental decline, and can help reduce the risk of age-related Alzheimer's disease. Research has shown it may even help to lower blood pressure. Research has determined Vitamin C supplements reduce LDL (the bad) cholesterol and blood triglycerides. M 90 mg, W 75 mg *Smokers - add 35 mg*, UL 2000 mg

Vitamin D – A fat-soluble vitamin, all compounds of Vitamin D are produced in your skin when exposed to sunlight. There are also foods that contain Vitamin D, as well as supplements. Vitamin D was added to milk in the 1930s as a public health initiative to combat rickets (a disease that causes deformities and poor bone development in children) and continues to be an added nutrient to milk. Vitamin D has an especially important role as it regulates the absorption of phosphorus and calcium in your system, contributing to the growth of bones, teeth, and the immune system function. A lack of Vitamin D can produce soft bones (osteomalacia) or fragile bones (osteoporosis). Vitamin D has also been linked to improving symptoms of depression. If there is too much Vitamin D in your diet, be aware you may find your balance is affected as well as tendencies for kidney stones. Just keep an eye on your intake, adults of 3000 to 4000 IU per day, and you'll reap the wonderful benefits of Vitamin D. 30 to 70 years of age 15 mcg, 71+ 20 mcg, UL 50 mcg

Vitamin E (Alpha-tocopherol) – You may know Vitamin

E as an essential nutrient, containing anti-inflammatory properties and also as a powerful antioxidant that helps in repairing damaged cells. Vitamin E supplements can be found in topical products as well as oral supplements, aiding in the skin's suppleness and anti-aging appearances. With its ability to repair damaged cells, Vitamin E may even be beneficial at reducing internal damage to the skin, as in severe sunburn occurrence. Vitamin E is a fat-soluble essential nutrient and can be absorbed better when coupled with Vitamin C and is often found in multivitamin supplements. M 15 mg, W 15 mg (synthetic Vitamin E should be taken at approximately 10% increase), UL 1000 mg

Vitamin F – Not a vitamin in the common sense of the word, Vitamin F is a term for two fats, alpha-linolenic acid (ALA) an omega-3 fatty acid, and linoleic acid (LA) an omega-6 fatty acid, which is essential for certain brain and heart health functions, as well as aiding growth development, and reduced inflammation in joints and organs. Your brain is comprised of 60% fat, of which half is omega-3 fatty acids, that help in brain function, memory, and also contributes to staving off dementia and Alzheimer's disease. It was discovered in the 1920s that fat-free diets had horrible consequences on lab rats, later realizing what they had named as Vitamin F was in fact, these two key functioning fats. As these fatty acids are not produced in your body, they need to be included in your healthy and well-balanced diet. Deficiencies can show as dry skin, hair loss, slow wound healing, skin problems, and brain and vision defects. Supplements are offered as linoleic acid (LA) adult dosage at 11 – 16 grams per day and alpha-linolenic acid (ALA) 1.1 to 1.6 grams per day, and work in conjunction with each other to provide the best benefits.

Vitamin H (Biotin) – Vitamin H, or most currently referred to as Biotin, is among the B complex vitamin group and, along with many vitamin groups, helps your body convert food into energy. Though biotin, a water-soluble vitamin, is often linked to achieving shiny hair, strong nails, and improved skin, it is an essential nutrient for pregnant women and found in most prenatal vitamins as it helps in fetal development. Promoting a healthy liver is also on the list for its benefits. Though Biotin is most often consumed as a supplement taken in either capsule form or powder to add to shakes or smoothies, it is also available in a liquid. In its natural form, Biotin is found in eggs, cauliflower, mushrooms, spinach, cheeses, and almonds, though concentration is a bit low and if your diet isn't chock full of these foods, a supplement would definitely be your most convenient method of attaining its benefits. M 30 mcg, W 30 mcg

Vitamin K (Phylloquinone, Menadione) – This vitamin, a fat-soluble, plays a role in the clotting of the blood, namely by activating essential calcium and other proteins for the process. Vitamin K is essential in forming sphingolipids, a type of fat found densely packed into brain cells. This fat is also associated with improving episodic memory, which is the ability to absorb and remember verbal instructions. While it isn't necessary to take this vitamin as a standalone supplement, you may see it included in multivitamins. It can be found in many green vegetables, including broccoli, asparagus, okra, Brussel sprouts, frozen peas, and cabbage. *Caution: If you are taking Warfarin, talk to your medical provider as Vitamin K has detrimental reactions with this drug.* M 120 mcg, W 90 mcg

Chapter Summary

- Vitamins are organic-based and can lose their potency when exposed to heat or air.

• A lack of certain vitamins makes a body susceptible to many diseases, including scurvy, blindness, and rickets.

• Sufficient quantities of certain vitamins increase a body's health, such as having strong bones, healthy teeth, and prevention of birth defects.

IN THE NEXT CHAPTER, FACT SHARING IS LED BY THE minerals' role as a water-regulator.

CHAPTER FOUR: MINERALS

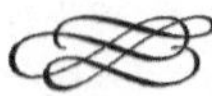

"*I read everything I could get my hands on about how the body reacts to competition, performance under stress, and the demon of fatigue. I learned how the body processes food when these conditions are present and what nutrients promote digestion, and aid in making this process flow smoothly.*

Then, I restructured the changes I needed to make in order to give my body the nutrients it required. I also needed to rethink how I could get the required nutrients to my necessary systems in a form which would be best utilized, under such strenuous conditions.

The answer … provide foods and nutrients which are easy for the body to process and absorb, thereby not making it work harder and get the essentials to their specific locations."

As the body doesn't manufacture minerals, we are entirely dependent on the food we consume to achieve the levels needed for health and wellbeing. Minerals and several precious metals, such as copper and iron, contribute to hundreds of necessary body functions. While balanced diets can supply some of these nutrients, supplementing minerals will guarantee needs are met so you can do activities without stress or injury and feel great while doing them.

When we think about all that is needed to get through a day, it's amazing we can even come close to what our bodies require. A hamburger here or a smoothie there can satisfy an instant need, but in the long run, how can we know just what is best for our body and what will cause it harm? Trusting ourselves to social media or the latest ad campaign can be risky, especially when we consider what their objective is. And it's probably not in our better interest!

Governing yourself to achieve a healthy body does take some effort and coordination. Minerals add to the picture in regulating and helping systems in your body build strength, which makes your job easier in planning a complete and well-balanced diet. Minerals also protect organs and support cardio, digestive, and neuro systems. While you will find the most common and effective minerals listed below, which will give you the needed building blocks for peak performance, a few not so popular minerals have been included. These can also be found in MVM's and may also play an important part in your overall well being, though they haven't been topping the popularity lists. All of these play important roles and should have a place in your diet.

Dosages are listed below as they were listed in the Vitamins chapter, with men (M) and women (W) considered as adult 19-year-olds unless otherwise stated. Upper limit dosage (UL) will follow if there is one available.

Calcium – One of the most widely understood minerals, due to marketing and government education programs, calcium builds and protects bones and teeth and helps with muscle dexterity. It also plays a part in blood clotting and nerve impulse communication. Sub-roles of calcium are seen in enzyme and hormone activity, as well as participation in maintaining healthy blood pressure. 31 to 50 years of age, M

1000 mg, W 1000 mg; 51 – 70 M 1000 mg, W 1200 mg; 71+ M 1200 mg, W 1200 mg; UL 2500 mg

Chloride – Balances fluids in the stomach, and are essential nutrients for digestion. Found in salt, soy sauce, and most processed foods. 14 to 50 years of age 2.3 g; 51 – 70 2.0 g; 71+ 1.8 g

Choline – This mineral helps neurotransmitter acetylcholine, assisting brain and nerve activity. It also helps metabolize fats and their movement and is found in milk, eggs, organ meats, and peanuts. M 550 mg, W 425 mg, UL 3500 mg

Chromium – A key nutrient in the maintenance of insulin levels, chromium helps to balance blood glucose. This nutrient is essential in freeing energy from glucose. Most meats, fish, eggs, nuts and potatoes have measurable levels of chromium. Though it is found in several common dietary foods, quite often getting your required dosage through them often causes bloating. Those susceptible to acid reflux will find it particularly bothersome. Therefore, supplemental intake with a multivitamin and minerals will reduce these effects considerably. 14 to 50 years of age M 35 mcg; 14 to 18 years of age W 24 mcg; 19-50 W 25 mcg; 51+ M 30 mcg, W 20 mcg

Copper – Our immune systems rely heavily on essential nutrients and having copper in your arsenal is a wise decision. Copper balances iron metabolism as well as the immune system and helps create red blood cells. Though it is found in liver, shellfish, nuts, seeds, and whole grains, only about half of the nutrient is absorbed. M 900 mcg, W 900 mcg, UL 10,000 mcg

Fluoride – As a mineral, most of us know fluoride as an additive in our toothpaste and, depending on state regulation, is often added to our tap water. Fluoride helps build strong bones and fights cavity decay in teeth. It can also be found in some fish and tea. This mineral flushes through our system easily, though can be harmful to children if consumed in excessive amounts.

Iodine – It was found that iodine cannot be synthesized in our bodies in 1924, constituting the governments' request to add it to salt in the form of potassium iodide. Over the next 10 years, there was a notable fall in people with goiters from 30% to about 2%. Today, you will see salt being sold with iodine as well as without, though it is probably not necessary for addition to our diets now. Iodine is found in the thyroid hormone, contributing to body temperature. Iodine also contributes to nerve and muscle function, as well as growth and fertility. Congenital thyroid disorder is also prevented with iodine intake. M 150 mcg, W 150 mcg

Iron – Hemoglobin, found in red blood cells, is assisted by iron, to transport oxygen to muscles throughout the body. Along with helping myoglobin also, iron is needed to trigger chemical reactions, producing amino acids, neurotransmitters, hormones, and collagen. It can be found in red meat, poultry, green vegetables, and fortified grain products, but is found to be the most common supplement prescribed by medical professionals, particularly in women 15 to 50 (child-bearing years). 19 to 50 years of age M 8 mg, W 18mg; 51+ M 8 mg, W 8 mg

Magnesium – Chemical reactions depend on magnesium to work with calcium in muscle dexterity, blood clotting, and blood pressure policing. It also contributes to strengthening teeth and bones (where it is most often stored). Spinach, legumes, cashews, and seeds, as well as halibut and milk, contain magnesium, and you will always find it in multivitamin supplements.

Manganese – This mineral metabolizes carbohydrates and cholesterol, making it very popular in the 1980s when attention was focused on cardiovascular health. Manganese also assists in forming bones and balancing amino acids and can be found in fish, nuts, whole grains, and tea. While taking supplements containing manganese, watch levels, as some areas add this to drinking water, and those with liver conditions should monitor closely. M 2.3 mg, W 1.8 mg.

Molybdenum – Though deficiencies in molybdenum are rare, this key component of many enzymes helps to protect neurological systems in infants, which otherwise can lead to a particular form of infant mortality. It is a micronutrient that is essential for life and can be found in nuts, grains, milk, and legumes. M 45 mcg, W 45 mcg

Phosphorus – Assists in building and protecting teeth and bones and is found in DNA and RNA. While it also assists in converting food to energy, its main benefit moves nutrients in and out of cells. Even with ample doses of phosphorus, your body may still suffer from its lack, as some drugs adhere to it, disabling its effectiveness, which in turn causes bone loss, weakness, and even pain. Found in a wide variety of foods, such as dairy products, meat, fish, and poultry, a supplement will benefit most people and is found in most multivitamin supplements. M 700 mg, W 700 mg, UL 31 to 70 years of age, 4000 mg; 71+ 3000 mg

Potassium – Potassium works in the fluids within our bodies and is needed to keep muscles agile and supple. While it also helps to maintain steady heart rhythm and nerve impulses, studies have found its presence also lowers blood pressure. It is thought to also contribute to bone mass. Monitor this nutrient, as high doses may be toxic to your system – intake of meat, milk, fruits, and vegetables contain potassium, but overconsumption of supplementals is usually what triggers higher levels. Keep to the suggested numbers here, and you'll have balanced and sustainable levels. M 4.7 g, W 4.7 g

Selenium – This mineral acts as an antioxidant and

balances unstable molecules which can cause cell damage. It also contributes to balancing thyroid hormone activity. Studies are being conducted to see if it has the potential to lower the risk of certain cancers, but nothing has been conclusive. Selenium can be found in organ meats, seafood, and walnuts. M 55 mcg, W 55 mcg, UL 400 mcg

Sodium – Regulates the fluids in the body and assists in nerve impulses. Muscles benefit from sodium also, as it aids in contraction responses. Medical physicians recommend limited doses of sodium, as it can lead to increased blood pressure, and suggest a limit of consumption to 2300 mg per day. However, average consumption usually ranges between 4000 and 6000 mg per day. Be sure to regulate this intake, as it can also lead to water retention, muscle fatigue, and general overall sluggishness. It is found in salt, soy sauce, and processed foods. M 2300 mg, W 2300 mg

Sulfur – While sulfur aids to form bridges between different protein structures and is needed for healthy hair, skin, and nails, there is no recommended dosage for its benefit. It is a component of thiamin and certain amino acids and can be found in protein-rich foods.

Zinc – Zinc plays a key role in the body, as it allows Vitamin A to be released from the liver, and is needed to help build the immune system, form enzymes, and build cell regeneration. Studies have shown zinc, when combined with some antioxidants, may delay age-related progress of macular degeneration in the eyes. Though found most often in red meats and oysters, it can also be found in fortified cereals, beans, and nuts. Supplemental additions are beneficial in most instances, especially for vegetarians, as it is found in lesser degrees in a plant-based diet. M 11 mg, W 8 mg

CHAPTER SUMMARY

• Minerals are inorganic nutrients that hold on to their chemical base. This means they can be found in many of the foods we eat and keep their potency throughout processing.

• Minerals can be categorized into major, minor, and trace elements.

• Many of the major minerals are stored in the body.

IN THE NEXT CHAPTER, DISCOVER HOW MANY EVERYDAY remedies are actually made from herbs.

CHAPTER FIVE: BOTANICALS AND HERBS

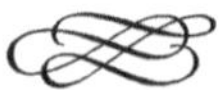

"When I changed the method of food and supplement intake during competition, my entire world changed. Because I reduced the strain on my digestive system of processing the food I consumed, I reduced the enzymes and amino acids needed to break the food down. Those enzymes and amino acids could then go to other needed areas in my body which took a back seat to the immediate need of energy and stamina during competition, not to mention supporting my systems which produced adrenaline.

Adrenaline also plays a part of good guy/bad guy, a bit like caffeine does in our bodies when we need a boost. It's great for the initial kick when we begin a workout or physical event, but in the long run, it overworks the muscles and systems, reducing its effect, and production depletes the already strained systems from the activity."

Many lists of antioxidants exist, and include the beneficial claims of one or another and the benefits they may provide. The bottom line is this, many elements found in nature are beneficial to our bodies, such as green tea to promote digestive cleansing or mustard paste to soothe a bee sting. But for every one of the beneficial nutrients, it seems there are 5 others which aren't worth the bottle they're packaged in.

It is not this book's purpose to judge, but if a bet were to be placed on a category of bogus essential nutrients, botanicals and herbs would have the longest list, with antioxidants a close second. Manufacturers and marketers of these essentials are to blame, as the claims are usually exaggerated and state claims which are easily misinterpreted.

It is also true, many herbals are still being associated with their age-old myths and reputations - all the more reason to familiarize yourself with the ones that work and are helpful aids to your overall fitness and health.

In this chapter, you will find only beneficial elements, unless otherwise stated, as either something to couple with another nutrient or advice on governing its benefits due to its popularity. All botanical and herbal supplements are derived from plants and their many parts, roots, seeds, flowers, and the oil which is rendered from the plant.

Due to the fact that many people have sporadic success with certain herbs, in one instance it performs wonderfully and the next performance is less than desirable, other contributing factors are most likely affecting the success or failure, but also could be related to the age of the substance and the health of the plant at harvesting.

Descriptions here will peel away the assumptions of how and why certain botanicals and herbs work, their optimum storage needs (as many lose potency if not properly managed), and any necessary details or interactions you will want to know in order to make wise decisions about your health.

Because botanicals and herbs have been used for such a long time, new research and study findings are usually tied to medical advances on deciphering their elements or discovering new interactions between different elements. As our medical knowledge expands, so does our ability to use these supplements in their most advantageous and specific ways. Many athletes and non-athletes alike are taking advantage of the benefits. The Centers for Disease Control determined more than half of all Americans use herbal supplements.

- Botanical and herbal supplements can be used in many different forms
- Tablets and capsules
- Teas
- Liquid extracts
- Oils
- Bath salts
- Ointments

Generally, these supplements are safe to use, but people who are sensitive to plants or have allergies can have adverse reactions to many and should approach their use with caution. The FDA is responsible for consumer safety, but because many of these supplements were being manufactured and sold before 1994 when the Dietary Supplement Health Education Act was imposed, the monitoring is limited to reactionary and new labeling statements only. If botanicals and herbs have cautions or concerns, it is generally due to pre-existing conditions or pre-existing health issues in the person being treated with drugs. *Always* talk to a healthcare professional if you have questions about beginning an herbal supplement regimen.

Aloe vera - mostly used as a soothing skin topical, but has also been sold as a digestive aid for gastritis or constipation. When taken internally it lowers potassium levels. *Caution: If you take diuretics or digoxin, avoid taking aloe, because of its characteristics of altering of potassium levels.*

Astragalus (Astragalus membranaceus) - This herb reduces stress and was initially used in ancient Chinese medicinal practices. It is known to reduce oxidative stress and prevent cell damage while promoting the immune system.

Beta carotene - Known as an antioxidant, it fights free radicals (toxins which left unchecked, harm cells and body tissue). Though still widely used, studies have shown mixed carotenes prove to occasionally increase the chance of serious health risks. You will find substitutes for beta carotene (other carotenoids) in mixed and multiple compound supplements.

Black cohosh - This is a popular nutrient for menopausal discomforts including hot flashes, night sweats, and vaginal dryness. Available as a standalone or in multi-supplement tablets. *Caution: Do not take this in high levels or with antihypertensive medications, as it lowers blood pressure.*

Cannabidiol (CBD) - Recently, State and Federal regulation of some 'botanical' supplements have been under scrutiny, namely cannabidiol. While the government's position on CBD is confusing at best, due to the fact many who aren't educated on the origin of CBD, it is thought to create the sensation of being 'high'. CBD is derived from hemp, a cousin of marijuana, and does not create the lightheadedness and euphoria marijuana is known for. CBD has several health advantages, but none more strong than its effectiveness in treating child epilepsy, some forms of which there are no other known treatments. In fitness training and supplemental effectiveness, topical balms have many athletes swearing by its benefits. If ingested, however, uses focus on relief from anxiety and insomnia. New studies are now publishing success with help for chronic pain and arthritis (as a topical). It has been found to be safe, though it can react with blood thinners and has been known to cause nausea, fatigue, and irritability. The most obvious issue with CBD, however, is how the supplement is currently categorized. The FDA does not regulate the safety and purity of CBD, as it is sold as a supplement and not as a medication. Be cautious, as label statements for ingredients may not be entirely truthful and could contain elements unknown which may have adverse effects. Effective dosage for this supplement is also still unknown and potency of products is at the manufacturer's discretion. *If you do find a product that performs as claimed and intended, stay with the same manufacturer. Chances are good the batches will be consistent with ingredient potency and dose.*

Chamomile - Often used as a soothing tea to treat insomnia, chamomile has also gained awareness for anxiety, upset stomach, and several digestive maladies. Because it is a close cousin to ragweed, people who are allergic to ragweed should stay clear of chamomile.

Crocin - Found in saffron, Crocin is a yellow carotenoid pigment and has shown many health benefits in relation to anti-inflammatory, anti-anxiety, and antidiabetic effects. It has been studied as a protectant against age-related mental decline, by inhibiting the production of glycation end products (AGEs) and reactive oxygen species, linked to cell decline. It also helps to protect skin cells against UV-light-induced cellular damage, treatments used in several skin diseases.

Curcumin - As the main active compound in turmeric, curcumin has been attributed to have high antioxidant potential, and has shown to also possess anti-aging properties. It fights cell damage and activates many proteins, including sirtuins, which help delay cellular breakdown.

Echinacea - This helps to reduce symptoms of colds and flu. Though no scientific studies show echinacea prevents colds and flu symptoms, many people swear by its properties, with several over-the-counter products stating the benefits.

Ephedra (Ephedra sinica, Ma-Huang) - Used to treat

coughs and weight loss. *Caution: This herbal has many harmful interactions with heart medications and can be dangerous (even life-threatening), by raising heart rates and blood pressure.*

Epigallocatechin gallate (EGCG) - Impressive health benefits have been linked to EGCG, which is a concentrated polyphenol found in green tea. Research supports a reduction in several cancer risks and heart diseases. It is also known to possibly restore mitochondrial function in cells, which slows the aging process and increases the removal of damaged material in cells. Green tea and EGCG is associated with reduced incidence in diabetes, stroke, and heart disease. EGCG can also be ingested with supplements, in addition to green tea.

Feverfew (Tanacetum parthenium) Feverfew thins the blood, making it popular when trying to control migraines, arthritis, and some allergies. *Caution: Due to feverfews' blood-thinning qualities, blood clotting may be lessened, check with your medical professional before using.*

Flaxseed - Known for its beneficial content of omega-3 fatty acids and fiber, it is also a good source for lowering cholesterol.

Garlic (Allium sativum) - Long used as a preventative and treatment for colds, garlic has also shown it aids in clearing infections and lowering cholesterol. Its anti-inflammatory and anti-aging properties continue to gather attention in the research field and advances continue to be discovered. *Caution: If you are taking an anticoagulant, such as warfarin or Coumadin, excessive bleeding may occur. Contact your medical provider before use.*

Ginger - Ginger has a multitude of benefits, ranging from relief from nausea and motion sickness to lowering blood cholesterol and attacking free radicals. *Caution: It is a* *blood thinner, so caution should be used when taking other medications, consult your medical provider before using.*

Ginkgo - Ginkgo has long been used to help with memory loss, but more and more people are using it as an antidepressant because of its selective serotonin reuptake inhibitors (SSRIs). If you have side effects with antidepressant medications, you may want to try ginkgo; it also is known to help enhance sex drive and performance, though this has little scientific conclusions. An odd side note with ginkgo, it's been known to help tinnitus (ringing in the ears) also. *Caution: if you are taking blood thinners, heart medication, or prescription drugs, do not take ginkgo, as it alters the way your body processes medications.*

Ginseng (Panax ginseng) - Ginseng has been known to be an all-around beneficial botanical, which slows the aging process, boosts immunity, increases physical stamina and sexual performance, as well as mental capacity. *Caution: It should not be taken by people with high blood pressure.*

Goldenseal (Hydrastis Canadensis) - Because of its uses as an anti-inflammatory, constipation is eased with goldenseals use. *Caution: Because of its medicinal altering characteristics, it should be used with caution if you are taking any kind of heart or prescription medications.*

Green Tea - Though green tea is often referred to as 'The King' in antioxidant believers, it has many other benefits to your health. Considering its antioxidant advantages, it fights cell damage and attacks free radicals, it also increases the antioxidant capacity of the body. It also promotes heart health and shows reduction tendencies in LDL cholesterol by 4.5%. Green tea has shown to decrease blood pressure in obese people while helping with weight loss (containing both catechins and caffeine have shown to assist regulating hormones which promote weight reduction). Brain function increases with green teas' decrease of heavy metals element action, and improves connections in the brain, thereby improving functionality. While liver function hasn't been directly associated with green tea, it is also suspected it helps to decrease enzyme levels which improves liver health. Body systems are also found to recover quicker if green tea is consumed after exercise and physical stress related activities. The EGCG found in green tea also regulates the production of blood sugar, keeping levels low. Overall, it is easy to see why it is considered such a supplemental powerhouse. 250 to 500 mg per day and best when taken with food (as some find it to be acidic).

Hawthorn - (Crataegus species) The most notorious benefit of hawthorn treats congestive heart failure and high blood pressure. *Caution: due to its responsive nature, this should not be taken without advice from your medical physician.*

Licorice root (Glycyrrhiza glabra) - Often used for excessive coughs, cirrhosis, and digestive maladies, particularly with the stomach. *Caution: Licorice root raises blood pressure and should not be taken by anyone with a heart condition or on medication. Consult your medical professional if considering using it.*

Nettle (Urtica dioica) - Used to treat conditions in the lower digestive tract, such as urinary tract infection, bladder and kidney stones, and rheumatism. It is also found in many shampoos and conditioners as it helps control dandruff. *Caution: if you have trouble with your kidney or heart, consult with your medical provider before taking, as this will interfere with water and fluid retention.*

Peppermint oil - This has been used as a digestive aid for centuries and still is used to this day for such. Specifically treats nausea, indigestion, stomach problems, and bowel conditions. Many believe it clears the mind and brain fog when used in aromatherapy.

Rhodiola - Among the benefits Rhodiola is associated

with, anti-inflammatory and anti-aging top the list. It has led to increased life span in research and continues to be studied for other advantageous properties.

Soy - High cholesterol levels are lessened when taking soy, as well as increasing memory and lessening menopausal symptoms. Use organic, whole soy food as opposed to processed products, as the benefits are lessened after processing.

St. John's Wort - It has long been understood St. John's Wort treats depression, sleep disorders, and anxiety. *Caution: This herb has adverse interactions with many drugs. If you are taking any medications, consult a medical provider before using it.*

Tea tree oil - Well known healing agent to many skin conditions, including athlete's foot, nail fungus, wounds, infections, lice, thrush, acne, cold sores, and dandruff.

Turmeric - See above, Curcumin.

White willow bark - Known for its benefits in reducing pain, fever, and inflammation, it is the base plant derivative for aspirin. Can be purchased as a supplement tablet, salve, or extract.

NOTE: IF YOU ARE TAKING ANY KIND OF PRESCRIBED drug, such as digoxin, diuretics, hypoglycemics, nonsteroidal anti-inflammatory drugs, spironolactone, or warfarin, DO NOT use herbal supplements without first checking with your prescribing doctor. The botanicals and herbs which are known to cause reactions have been listed accordingly in the description and use, but your medical provider knows your body and its systems, and will be the best person to consult for your questions and concerns.

CHAPTER SUMMARY

- Herbs and botanicals have been made to support the human diet since time began.

- Most common herbal supplements are known for their pain-reducing and relief effects.

- Mixing herbs and botanicals can be beneficial, as well as harmful - knowledge is crucial.

IN THE NEXT CHAPTER, YOU WILL SEE HOW FREE radicals can affect a healthy body and what you can do to prevent it.

CHAPTER SIX: ANTIOXIDANTS

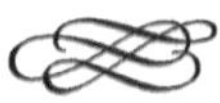

"*So, how did I reduce the strain of competition, still consume the foods and essential nutrients my body systems were dependent on, as well as achieve the results needed to win?*

I pureed my food, which assimilated the nutrients to easily-digested forms, easing the demands on my digestive system and quickening their absorption into my system. I also took all of my supplements in liquid form, which I highly recommend ... always. This gave me almost immediate availability of their benefits, which my body was in need while under stress.

I also began my recovery after each competition immediately with children's electrolyte liquids. These products contained specific easily digestible nutrients. Adult recovery liquids are harder on the system and can bog down the absorption of nutrients. When compared to the rate of absorption with the children's electrolyte liquids, adult liquids were almost 30% slower in getting to the needed parts of the body. Children's electrolyte liquids are the most digestible hydration available and a must for competitions and athletic exertion."

Although antioxidants have been studied for many years

in medical and biological studies and research, it is just in the past few decades that this term has become popular. The public has been bombarded with their need, and 'ignoring any incorporation of antioxidants into your diet will surely guarantee a toxic ravaged body' without any defenses or resilience.

Antioxidants inhibit the oxygenation of toxins in the body and are key components to preventing and destroying toxins and free radicals (the components attacking our body's cells). The waste our body produces from breaking down food and creating energy can be oxygenated, and when it is, it forms into free radicals and develops into chains, which attack healthy cells. Our bodies have always been fighting this internal battle, but now with the knowledge of antioxidants and their benefits, we can consume needed doses to eliminate free radicals and their dangers..

In the last few decades, the research being conducted on the effects of stress, smoking, sun exposure, and air pollution have on our bodies (namely research focused on artery-clogging diseases) has been intensified. Discovery of these modern-day conditions which create free radicals to a degree we have never known, brings the need for supplemental antioxidants to the forefront when planning a defense for your healthy diet and immune system regimen.

Antioxidants can be enzymes, which include many vitamins such as vitamins C and E. They can also be chemical compounds such as beta carotene or minerals such as manganese. There are thousands of different elements which can be described as an antioxidant. Naturally occurring antioxidants in our food are the basis of the natural defense in our systems. However, as you've read here, compounds can be changed in the body and the same is true for antioxidants.

If you single out one antioxidant to achieve all the benefits 'antioxidants' are claimed to achieve, you will be short-changed. Not all of them are rated equally effective, and just like the other supplements you've discovered here, each has its place in your diet.

Though research hasn't come to any radical conclusions about antioxidants' role in a thorough defense, it has shown us several areas where antioxidants are important in maintaining a healthy body . If partnered with other beneficial nutrients, antioxidants can play a key part in keeping your body strong, fit, and able to handle the challenges you ask of it daily.

How the marketing strategy on antioxidants began –

In 1991, the United States Department of Agriculture (USDA) created a scientific tool, the Oxygen Radical Absorbance Capacity (ORAC). Foods were rated and those high in antioxidants (the combatants of oxygenating toxins) were put in the spotlights, such as blueberries, cocoa, many spices, and legumes. These foods were promoted prominently as disease-fighters beginning with cancer and ending with heart disease. Even benefits were listed for brain health and functionality.

As time progressed, however, the USDA has withdrawn the information, because many antioxidants are not directly involved with free radicals. The hype was quieted, but the idea is still very prominent in the marketing and selling of antioxidants.

The largest fact realized in antioxidant trials and research is this – no antioxidant by itself will rid the body of the free radicals (which contribute to heart disease) or can eliminate toxins (which build your resistance to cancer).

What has been determined is this – by combining antioxidants with other combative nutrients, they can be valuable in reducing accumulations of toxins and free radicals. It has also been determined antioxidants work best when consumed through natural foods instead of artificially produced supplements, needing about half of the dose as an artificially produced antioxidant. For some reason, they respond, absorb, and eliminate toxins and free radicals easily and in greater quantity, when digested in their natural form and are supported by their natural 'helper' nutrients. As our body processes natural foods easily, any substance that is artificial is harder for the digestive system to assimilate and gather nutrients from.

The recent years of marketing antioxidants has shown how easily a term can be misunderstood. When we see 'antioxidant' listed on a green tea or fortified cereal, we believe it will benefit our well-being and naturally choose this product over another which doesn't list this benefit. Though antioxidants are beneficial, rarely are they in a form in processed consumables which would actually assist in eradicating free radicals in our system. When you are aware of the leniency manufacturers take when packaging their products, you can make better decisions about what is actually contained in the foods you eat and if the claims are just for show or actually do what they advertise.

With that in mind, let's explore the most beneficial antioxidants and the natural foods they are found in to supplement your diet and fitness plan. All foods are at their peak and highest beneficial value when consumed fresh, and not processed (frozen, cooked, or canned) and are listed here with this in mind, unless otherwise noted.

Anthocyanins - This group of antioxidants are found in deeply colored fruits, such as blueberries and purple grapes. These compounds, with anti-inflammatory effects, fight against oxidative stress and inflammation, which have both been attributed to brain aging and neurodegenerative diseases. Accumulations of anthocyanins have also shown to improve communication between neurons and other brain cells when processing information and are attributed to help to clear brain fog.

Beta-carotene, other carotenoids, and lycopene – Though beta-carotene can be harmful if consumed in excessive amounts, if you are aware of what you are eating and do not overindulge, it will be of benefit to your fitness diet plan. Studies have shown carotenoids and lycopenes can provide similar benefits with little risk to existing serious health issues. They have slowly been replacing beta carotenes' role in supplements, though they are still prevalent and highly sought after in most nutritional fitness planning. Foods where you'll find these beneficial compounds include apricots, asparagus, beets, broccoli, cantaloupe, carrots, bell peppers (all colors), kale, leafy greens (collard, spinach, and turnip), mangos, oranges, peaches, pink grapefruit, pumpkin (unprocessed and without sugar), squash (winter), sweet potato, tangerines, tomatoes, and watermelon.

Coenzyme Q10 (CoQ10) - Your body produces this antioxidant. As you age, it's levels decrease, making cells vulnerable to damage from outside elements as well as free radicals inside your system. CoQ10 has been known to reduce physical and mental deterioration, as well as oxidative stress (a phenomenon that occurs inside the body and is an accumulation of free radicals and other elements that accelerate aging and age-related diseases).

Fisetin - Known as a flavonoid compound, it is considered a senotherapeutic. It reduces cells which, due to irregular composition, decline and deteriorate, causing cells to expire. Fisetin eradicates this process.

Flavonoids - These antioxidant plant compounds are prevalent in dark chocolate and are found in the parts of the brain associated with learning and memory. It is also thought that flavonoids help slow age-related mental decline, while also contributing to memory retention. Mood boosting has also been associated with the flavonoids found in dark chocolate, though the taste may be playing into the scenario, just a bit.

Phenolic compounds – Included in these antioxidant compounds, phenols consist of hydroxyl structures which are both simple and complex. They include flavonoids, polymerics, tannins, and several other compounds of different classes. They are most prevalent and easily obtained in apples, red wine, and onions (as quercetin), berries, cocoa, and tea (as catechins), berries, grapes, peanuts, and red and white wine (as resveratrol), berries and spices (as coumaric acid), blueberries and strawberries (as anthocyanins).

Resveratrol - This polyphenol is found in the skin of grapes, berries, peanuts, and in red wine, and activates our bodies genes called sirtuins. It promotes cell longevity and lifespan, increasing resistance to disease and toxins.

Selenium – You read about this mineral previously in this book. You will see it mentioned often in multivitamin and mineral supplements too, though its most beneficial form of antioxidants are in fresh foods. They include beef, barley, Brazil nuts, brown rice, fish, and shellfish (crab, lobster, and shrimp).

Theanine (L-theanine) - Found in many teas, including green tea, theanine is also an amino acid and protects the function in neuro and brain function, extending cognition and awareness.

Vitamin C – You already know of the powerhouse attributes this vitamin supplies. Consume the following foods which are high in Vitamin C to benefit from the antioxidants. Vitamin C is found within broccoli, Brussels sprouts, cantaloupe, cauliflower, grapefruit, leafy greens (beet, collards, mustard, and turnip), honeydew, kale, kiwi, lemons, oranges, papaya, snow peas, strawberries, sweet potatoes, tomatoes, and all colors of peppers.

Vitamin E – Though Vitamin E can be absorbed in several forms, here we are referring to consumption through eating, as opposed to topical applications. Included are almonds, avocados, Swiss chard, leafy greens (beet, mustard, and turnip), peanuts, red peppers, spinach (boiled), and sunflower seeds.

Zinc – Again, you have read of the other benefits of zinc. It is found in its natural form in beef, cashew, chickpeas, fortified cereals, lentils, oysters, poultry, pumpkin seeds, sesame seeds, and shrimp, and provides antioxidant benefits for circulatory and digestive systems.

CHAPTER SUMMARY

• An antioxidant is a general term when referring to many compounds known to attach to and destroy toxins and free radicals.

• Free radicals are unstable or distorted molecules that damage cells and their membranes, located in all types of cells, such as DNA.

• Antioxidants can be found in many common foods and are best ingested in their natural forms.

IN THE NEXT CHAPTER, YOU WILL UNCOVER THE ROLE OF live probiotics in your digestive system.

CHAPTER SEVEN: PROBIOTICS, WEIGHT LOSS, AND FEELING GREAT

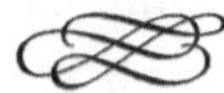

"*By the time the next major competition arrived, I had been able to implement and test my theory. I was also able to improve elements that proved to be challenging. After speaking with many like-minded athletes and colleagues, I also learned how baby food can play a key role in easily digestible yet incredibly nutritious consumables, as well as drinking liquids and gels to lessen the impact on my digestive tract and ease the absorption of essential nutrients into my system..*

I focused on the 2007 Nationals and World Championships to ultimately put my tried and true game plan to the test ..."

One of the first things we picture in our minds when we hear the word 'fitness' is a healthy trim, and well-functioning body, whether it's our own body or a distant picture from our middle school health class. Being fit requires many systems to run well, which in turn, support other body systems, thereby all contributing to a high performing machine.

As we've already talked about, our diet, what we consume in food and liquids, governs these systems' performance. If we eat well-balanced meals and snacks, our body will respond in kind and step up to the demands of fending off stressful situations, eliminate the chance of harmful diseases, or progress to a physical achievement requiring extended stamina and strength.

When we discuss probiotics, we are talking about the bacteria and microbes found in our digestive tract, or 'gut', which keep it healthy. Breaking down food into energy, which the bloodstream carries to various parts of our body, is its main function but there are many additional functions of the digestive system, and each task has particular needs to help in the overall process of turning food into energy..

Though there are several other parts of our body which contribute to the digestive process, we will concentrate here on the organs directly associated with probiotics.

The stomach, which has incredibly acidic enzymes, is the first level of processing food before it is passed along to the small intestine. It can also supply the bloodstream with liquids, especially if tissues are dehydrated or lacking nutrients. High energy packets and water-based glycerides can be digested here and passed on to needed cells, while solid foods continue on to the small intestine for further digestion.

In the small intestine, probiotics really begin their work. Food that isn't absorbed here moves to the large intestine. Waste which isn't used moves to the rectum, and is finally eliminated through the bowels.

Many people, including some medical professionals, believe most maladies begin in your gut. Allergies, auto-immunity, headaches, migraines, acne, skin rash, weight gain, yeast infections, fatigue, immune challenges, hormonal imbalances and even neuro-sensory, can be related to how healthy or unhealthy your gut is.

Your 'gut flora', or good and bad bacteria and microbes, can become unbalanced when your diet is poor and in need of vital nutrients, and imbalances can lead to what's known as a 'leaky gut'.

When you have a leaky gut, food particles and toxins escape through the tract lining and gut wall. When these particles are released into the body where they shouldn't be, they cause havoc, leading to an immune response and chronic inflammation. And that is where the real trouble begins, disrupting hormone imbalances, poisoning unarmed organs, and producing unhealthy systems.

One known reaction to leaky gut and hormone imbalance disrupts the estrobolome gut bacteria which metabolizes estrogens. By developing an imbalance, it increases the chance of early menopause, or eventually, postmenopausal breast cancer.

Further studies of an unhealthy gut have shown it can severely impact the nervous system, causing anxiety, depression, autism, and schizophrenia. This is because the digestive system creates almost all of the serotonin your body produces, up to 90%. Serotonin is the brain hormone which contributes to the feeling of happiness and wellbeing.

In addition to serotonin, your gut also produces over 30 neurotransmitters. Which only goes to prove, a digestion system which runs well keeps the rest of the body feeling well too!

Along with keeping your spirits up, serotonin contributes to keeping your bowels, heart, and bones 'happy' too. Not having enough serotonin will leave these body parts vulnerable and susceptible to irritable bowel syndrome, cardiovascular disease, and osteoporosis.

Modern diets, particularly in North America, rarely have a nutrient-rich balance, and therefore produce negligent effects on your digestive tract. Be aware of the nutrients contained in your favorite foods, as well as ones you plan on incorporating into your diet. By incorporating the needs of your gut flora into your diet plan, supplemental nutrients will improve your wellbeing. This in turn, makes you feel great and provides ample immune qualities that eliminate the chance of disease caused by imbalances. All systems benefit from essential nutrients that combat depression, disease, and chronic illnesses.

The digestive tract seems like a very large system to keep running smoothly and supporting the rest of the body's functions. Because of the fine balance needed to keep it healthy and working well, it seems near impossible to eat the right foods and supplements to maintain this fine balance. This is especially troubling when we consider how easy it is to pick up processed foods at the store, which may initially cut down on prep time, but in the long run, give little nutritional benefit to our body.

You may be feeling like a system which influences so much of a body's well being is next to impossible to keep healthy, but this isn't always the case. Even when a gut is out of balance and is the cause for chronic symptoms, it isn't impossible to get your digestive tract balanced again. But it may take a bit of time.

Due to the fact your diet plays such a big part in keeping your gut flora balanced, a few strategies in diet planning and supplements need to be taken, which can begin to change with your very next meal.

- Avoid artificial sweeteners. Even if you need that bit of 'sweet' in your meal, processed sugar has proven to be less harmful than artificial sweeteners.

- Magnesium is a good example of a needed mineral which is often found low or absent in healthy guts. By incorporating this mineral in your diet, you will be supplying much needed nutrients against imbalances and depressive symptoms.

• Fermented and cultured foods are gaining more and more popularity as healthy foods, but often, are falsely labeled. Make sure they are referring directly to the contents and not just a general statement, before giving them credit for being beneficial. Microorganisms which support your gut flora are yogurt (look for natural fermentation), sauerkraut, kombucha, and kimchi for optimal sources.

• By eliminating processed and inflammatory foods and oils, like cookies, chips, and vegetable oil, you will avoid many gut diseases. Not only is leaky gut avoided, but Crohn's disease can be sidestepped, and ulcerative colitis. Even so-called 'healthy' foods which have agave-sweetener in them can be bad choices. Instead, increase anti-inflammatory foods like non-starchy vegetables, like spinach and green beans, and wild-caught fish, which normalize levels and heal the tract.

• We've already discussed the benefits of antioxidants, and why are they so good? Because they attack free-radicals, which also like to live in your gut, damaging the lining walls. By adding colorful polyphenols, like berries, to your gut flora, your microbe balance will improve. Creating an antioxidant balance also builds defenses against many other diseases in the body, including once again, cancer and cardiovascular disease.

• Cortisol, or supplemented nutrients for cortisol replacement, alleviates the imbalances that lead to insulin resistance and deficiency in fighting stress. Anything which helps with neutralizing stress and its demons will benefit most systems in your body.

• Add fiber to your diet. Fiber gets fermented in your large intestine, which then turns into energy. Dietary fiber also supplies energy to your colon keeping it operating at an optimum functionality. Begin by adding cruciferous and leafy vegetables, berries, seeds, and raw nuts.

• Prebiotics are a type of fiber and are a food source for probiotics. Though finding natural foods with prebiotics in them may be a challenge, incorporating them into your diet is close to mandatory. Focus on cooked onion, asparagus (small amounts) as well as raw chicory root, Jerusalem artichoke and raw dandelion greens (large amounts).

With a list as long as this, and definitely longer when considering all needs of the gut, it is often a daunting task to assemble a well-thought-out and balanced diet to support all the probiotics your digestive tract needs. Often, a supplemental probiotic alternative helps to fill in needed essential nutrients.

Finally, if you have problems with blood sugar levels or high glucose, probiotics have shown to improve or control glycemic imbalance. This further leads to helping the body avoid insulin resistance, obesity, diabetes, and cardiovascular disease.

When choosing a probiotic, make sure it can go the distance. If your supplements don't make it to your intestines, they do little to help your imbalances. Because they are living creatures, probiotics need to be alive when ingested. Check the shelf life or expiration date as well as a statement on the label which mentions reaching your digestive tract. If they are consumed in the stomach, they will be of little benefit.

Also, make sure there are prebiotics in your supplement.

The probiotics need a bit of nourishment too, in order to perform the balancing act your gut flora needs and prebiotics are what nourishes and keeps the probiotics alive.

A final word on basic health which keeps your digestive tract in check and helps to promote balanced nutrients -

First, get plenty of sleep. Supplements can't do it all, so make sure they have a good base to work from. By having a body which has plenty of rest, you will decrease stress and anxiety, promote wellbeing, and avoid altering the good bacteria in your digestive tract.

Secondly, if you've developed chronic diseases or illnesses, taking a probiotic won't alleviate your condition. If more radical means are needed, don't rely on your probiotics to solve all problems. By balancing your gut flora, however, you will see severe cases lessen their symptoms, making a group assault on your illness more successful. Find answers to the other conditions you may need to address to achieve total health.

If you suspect an underlying condition, consult a health-care professional. They can run tests that will show deficiencies or other imbalances, giving you the information you need to plan your diet and eat wisely.

Chapter Summary

- Probiotics, such as bacteria and yeasts, provide digestive benefits.

- For probiotics to be beneficial, the microorganisms must be alive, as in yogurt.

- Probiotics are a new concept in dietary supplements - many manufacturers' labels can be misleading in their description, as the term hasn't been defined for consumer packaging by any government agency.

In the next chapter, you will learn how MVM's have played a major part in the nutritional evolution for the past 80 years.

CHAPTER EIGHT: MULTIPLE VITAMIN-MINERAL SUPPLEMENTS AND ESSENTIALS YOU SHOULDN'T MIX

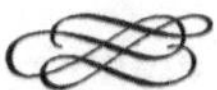

"Training had gone well, I felt lean and strong. My senses were keen and my thoughts focused. I could tell several of the competitors in my division were tense and, what looked like to be, unprepared. I reminded them we trained for this and all we have to do is follow our plan and remember our training.

Knowing I had crossed off all the boxes of eating right, fine-tuning my skills and building strength and agility to the best I'd ever achieved gave me the confidence and desire to move forward and face my opponents with assurance."

Multivitamins with Minerals are the people's favorite, accounting for close to one-sixth of all dietary supplements and 40% of all vitamins and mineral sales in the United States. To assume these are the best supplements to balance your diet would be a huge mistake, however.

In 1940, the first multivitamin and mineral supplements became available. Since then, many people have found convenience and reliability in their choice. They feel great, they only have to take one pill, and because they have been taking it over a long period of time, they trust the product to do as it promises.

But do they?

When manufacturers combine vitamins and minerals in their supplements, they are not regulated by any health or government agency. Levels of each essential nutrient can vary widely, as can the dosage of the nutrients. Though most are based on the RDA's suggestions, due to the lack of regulations, many are just nice packages wrapped up in deceiving labeling.

When you look at a multivitamin and mineral supplement, or MVM, they are required to list certain criteria of the ingredients. They must be listed in highest amount of content to least amount, and if an ingredient is a combined compound, all ingredients within that compound must also be listed, again, from highest to lowest amount contained.

If there is another name the nutrient is known as, you will see the name listed also, as in Vitamin A (as Retinyl Acetate) or Vitamin E (as di-Alpha Tocopheryl Acetate). You will also notice the percentages are listed under 'Daily Value' and usually referenced at the bottom of the label such as 'Based on a 2000 calorie Diet' or 'Daily Value not established'.

Because there will also be other ingredients which are in an MVM but have no sufficient nutritional value, they will be listed as 'Other Ingredients' such as corn syrup, sugar, or gelatin.

It's not to say just because a manufacturer can be devious means that they are. In the 21st century, we consumers have become much more aware of the ingredients in our consumables than we were 20 years ago. Many of us do read the labels, and are becoming more and more educated on the things which should be in the product, as well as some that shouldn't.

You are here reading this book, for instance, because you want to make sure what you are consuming is optimal for your body. And so, the manufacturers are balancing the walk on the fence with giving you the product you want while still keeping costs for manufacturing minimal.

Proof of the popularity of MVM's are all around us. At the grocery and drug counters, isle's are bursting with choices for MVM's as well as individual supplemental vitamins and minerals. Not only do we see vitamins and minerals, but products can also contain some of the previous chapter products of antioxidants, probiotics, and fitness supplements. They come in pill, liquid, powder, and chewable form.

What's best for you?

In order to make wise decisions about MVM supplements, you'll be using the same analogy as you have with the individual ones (as discussed in previous chapters). There is one happy reason which may sway you to the MVM team, and that is *convenience.*

But it's not just convenience in the sense that you don't have to buy bottle after bottle of individual nutrients. If your MVM has been formulated correctly, you also have the benefit of not combining nutrients that counteract each other or cause harm.

Another benefit of an MVM is choosing one which it targeted for your specific needs. If you are a senior woman over 50, there is an MVM section especially for you. If you are pregnant or have a child of 4, 8, or 12 years old, another shelf or two is devoted to your needs. You'll even be able to purchase MVM's which are formulated specifically for you if you want to control your weight, manage menopause symptoms, or improve your immune system.

Other specialties focus on specific multiples such as relief of joint pain or improved bone structure. And you may even see these combined with herbal or botanical supplements with specialty ingredients for skin firmness with coenzyme Q10 or gut health which include probiotics.

There are also packeted MVM's which contain several different pills to be taken together. Most of these are targeted at a specific consumer, perhaps high energy, antioxidant, athlete, or pregnant women. Others may be combined to achieve a particular function for improving your immune system, managing menopausal symptoms, or easing anxiety.

We've discussed a few of the combinations which are harmful in the vitamin and mineral chapters.

For instance, don't take zinc, magnesium, or calcium at the same time. Following is a list of combinations of vitamins and minerals, as well as a few drugs, you should avoid combining.

Antibiotics and Iron - Any antibiotic, especially those in the tetracycline family, will be affected by iron. It interferes with the antibiotics absorption, thereby reducing the effectiveness and intended benefits.

Antidepressants and St. John's wort - Both of these supplements increase the level of serotonin, the brain chemical which triggers happy feelings. But when taken together, they can cause fever, anxiety and confusion and lead to muscle rigidity and seizures (serotonin syndrome). Don't mix together.

Cimetidine (Tagamet HB) - This is a treatment for duodenal ulcers, and can slow the removal of caffeine from the body. Side effects from caffeine can be increased.

Diabetes medication and CoQ10 - CoQ10 is a powerful heart medicine. It also lowers blood sugars, which, if taken with other diabetes drugs, risks low levels of blood sugars. Because CoQ10 can also lower blood pressure, this combination can present dangerous low blood pressure and dizziness. If you have been taking them both, stop immediately. Even if you haven't had any symptoms, you can develop the risks without notice.

Fish oil and Ginkgo biloba - Ginkgo biloba (and garlic) are blood thinners, which are good reasons to take, as they improve your brain functions of memory and discourage headaches. But if you are in need of omega3's and are taking fish oil supplements, pairing these together could cause uncontrolled bleeding. Split them up by at least 2 to 3 hours between consuming for safety. If you are concerned or are taking blood thinners, consult a healthcare professional before taking fish oil supplements.

Garlic and OTC or Rx blood thinners - This warning was listed above, but you can't ever list cautions too many times. Garlic is a natural blood thinner, and if taken with any kind of blood thinner (Coumadin, warfarin), or even a baby aspirin, it can affect clotting and internal bleeding. Make sure your healthcare provider knows you are interested in adding garlic to your diet. Other natural essential nutrients which increase blood thinning are Vitamin E, Ginkgo biloba, fish oil, ginger, feverfew, and willow bark.

Iron and Green Tea - Mixing tea, black or green or curcumin supplements will defer any absorption of iron for at least 2 hours. Iron helps to distribute oxygen. If this is the main reason you are supplementing iron into your diet, be careful to not drink or consume these nutrients unless there is a 2 hour window or more between use.

Calcium and Potassium - When combined together, you will get less of each of these nutrients, as they affect each other's assimilation rate. You will notice, however, they are often suggested to take together, as both help the body absorb potassium. This can be lost if you exercise or are phys-ically active in humid climates. Take them about 4 hours or more apart to reap the benefits of each.

Magnesium and Calcium - Taking minerals together

may reduce the effectiveness or reduce the absorption of each. Take them at different times, perhaps one in the morning and one in the evening. If you have kidney or heart problems, it is best to take magnesium with a healthcare provider's knowledge, and always take on a full stomach and add a glass of water also. Some suggest taking magnesium before bed will help relax your body for a better nights' sleep.

Melatonin and other sedating herbs - Sedative herbs and supplements are easily overused. These include melatonin, St. John's wort, valerian, kava, and ashwagandha. Don't mix any of these together, as the effect may cause unexpected drowsiness. Often, there is a warning on the label of nutrients which are specific to each and what to anticipate from them.

Niacin and Red Yeast Rice - Both of these supplements are known as natural ways you may be able to lower your cholesterol. By using both of these, you can do harmful damage to your liver. Pick one or the other, but don't combine hoping for an 'increased benefit'. It will be increased harm instead.

Vitamins A, D, E, and K - All of these vitamins are fat-soluble, meaning they are stored in your body (the liver) before use in the body. In multivitamins, the levels of combination are most often desirable. But if you take them separately, take the Vitamin K 2 hours after taking any of the other vitamins. Vitamin K interferes with the absorption of many nutrients, including these vitamins and in a MVM, it isn't always wise to combine them in one dose..

Vitamin K and blood-thinning drugs - High blood pressure drugs and blood-thinning drugs can act severely with other nutrients, even many popular food items that counteract their function, such as broccoli, chickpeas, kale, and lettuce. Even echinacea, popular for easing cold symptoms, can decrease the effectiveness of blood thinners, to the point of risking a stroke. Do not mix any of these foods with Vitamin K in them when you are on blood thinners, such as warfarin or Coumadin.

Zinc and Copper - Zinc interferes with the absorption of copper into your system. If you need to take them both, 2 hours in between doses is sufficient. Also, taking zinc over a long period of time can deplete your copper levels and cause deficiency. Talk to your healthcare professional if you have low levels of copper in your system.

CHAPTER SUMMARY

- Multivitamins have been available to consumers since the 1940s.

- About 35% of all Americans take multivitamins.

- There are no regulations for what must be contained in a multivitamin and mineral supplement.

IN THE NEXT CHAPTER, LABELING AND DEFINITIONS WILL give you the needed information to make a wise choice when considering which supplements to incorporate in your diet plan.

CHAPTER NINE: MYTHS

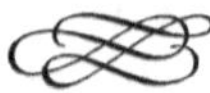

"*The final competition. I had successfully won four matches in the 2007 National Competition and this was for the final gold medal match. Facing my opponent as we were being introduced, I felt calm, confident, and quite excited to see how I would fare against this challenger.*

The rounds passed and with each match, I felt more confident and more in control. It wasn't that my body was running on a zealous level of anarchy, but rather, I didn't feel diminished in any way. My body reacted in the way I was asking it to, my head was clear with strategy and advantages, and I felt in sync with my continued strength, as my opponent began to become more aggressive. But there was one more final test ..."

Over the years, decades, and millennia, man has changed our ideas of what is healthy to eat, what is not, what foods weigh us down, and other products to consume without abandon.

Bananas have received a bad rap, as well as eggs and avocados. Even whole grains have a good and bad place in our diets.

But through all these ups and downs of what is good and

what isn't, several need to be addressed which are very good for our body and its systems, yet still are labeled as containing compounds which either present a direct detrimental risk to our health or may cause problems in the near future we will need to correct.

Below, you will read about several of these foods and supplements. There are more, to be sure, and as science and research learns of these discoveries, a well-informed and smart athlete will keep updated as these studies unfold.

Bagels - Many of us became hooked on bagels back in the 1990's, with more choices and availability seeping into the 2000s, up to today. Their popularity not only increased our love for breads, but it also increased our caloric intake, and most times, not with the best of carbs. Many, however, have found short-cuts to make this beloved food item beneficial to our nutritious diet and satisfy our craving for a much-loved food. Here are some ways to rethink your bagel desires.

Cut it in Half - Because most bagels are large enough to fill a backpack, the calorie count is off the charts. When you consider the shelf life of the bagel, usually a day or two, the temptation to eat the entire thing often wins out. Try eating just half of the bagel, either splitting it with a friend or finding a tight plastic container to save it for tomorrow's pleasure.

Remove the Innards - Perhaps you really want to eat the whole bagel - well, take out the inside, soft bread. You'll be removing just over half of the calories while still keeping the well-loved chewy and flavorful goodies found on the outside.

Whole-grain Options - While most bagels are known as a white flour, yeasty treat, many specialty bakeries have numerous options, including wheat, seeded, sprouts, and more. The choice for these options is less at the local market, so seek out individual locations for whole-grain choices galore.

Include Proteins - While there are carbs in every bagel, by putting tasty proteins on, and in, them, you can round out a great meal and not feel the extra carbs and possible fats. Try turkey and avocado, Neufchatel cheese and tomato, or spinach and salmon on your next bagel. Eggs and any nut butters are also tasty and nutritious choices, while balancing out blood sugars too.

Vegetables - Last, but certainly not least, put some vegetables together and load them on your bagel. Saute eggplant, turnips, tomatoes, or zucchini in a bit of olive oil for just a moment, and pile them onto your hollowed out bagel. Maybe even add in an egg for added protein. Leafy greens can also add some pep to your carb- they are easy, and if you gather sprouts and cottage cheese, you are set with great taste and essential nutrients and protein.

Cheese - If you were sad to see the effect some cheeses have on your system and had to be eliminated, fear not. There are several balanced and nutritious choices. Consider, by having a cheese which isn't laden with fats, you will also be adding calcium, protein, and Vitamin D, as well as many other beneficials, which you'll be happy by incorporating in your diet plan. If you take a closer look, the nutritious elements in cheese can outweigh the extra fat, and will give you a key diet food full of nourishment. Here are several with their benefits and advantages.

Cottage Cheese - Within the plastic container of a cheese you've known since childhood, you will find a plethora of casein protein, needed for muscle recovery. Many other proteins are included to aid in protein synthesis and absorption. When you add cottage cheese to fruit, such as cantaloupe, grapefruit, mangoes, or even tomatoes, a half-cup can give you 16 grams of protein for a satisfying snack or after workout boost. It is also a great additive to yogurt to increase satisfaction and proportions.

Feta - This cheese originated in the Mediterranean, but has long since been loved the world over. It is available in block or crumbled form and has a distinctive and slightly pungent aroma, which will give you the craving you may have without having to consume a large portion. It is on the lower end of calories, about 75 per ounce, and is traditionally made from goat's milk, but can be found made with other animals' milk, such as milk from cows.

Goat Cheese - Recently, this cheese has made a huge impact on the food market. In the last ten years, it has grown from a simple appetizer cheese paired often with fruit because of its mild sweetness, to being used in layered meat Wellington and fondue. It is lower on the caloric scale, just like Feta, and is loaded with many more nutrients. There is even enough protein in this cheese to supplement your diet with one entire serving. It can be paired with beets in salads and nuts, as well as crumbled on soups or oatmeal. It can often be substituted for cream cheese with fewer calories to justify.

Neufchatel - Originally produced in France, this American cream cheese cousin has found a loyal crowd, replacing many recipes straight across. With ⅓ fewer calories, it also scores high, and can be used in dips or spread on crackers and whole-grain breads as a recovery food after workouts.

Parmesan - If you are prone to stuff an omelet with cheddar or American cheese, try using parmesan next time. You will get a wonderful taste from the pairing of eggs and parmesan, as well as cutting back on unwanted fats, at 112 calories per ounce. As you get used to using this cheese, you will see it pairs well with many foods you may currently consume, such as grating some for adding on popcorn (instead of butter and salt) and shaving or shredding to top salads (use with a simple olive oil to lessen unwanted processed dressing ingredients).

Provolone - Put a slice of this cheese on a sandwich, and you will be adding a low-fat option, boosting the protein level once again, while at the same time, giving you some creamy satisfaction. By replacing cheddar, Swiss, or American cheese with Provolone, you will give yourself 21 percent of your recommended daily value of calcium too.

Ricotta - In addition to goat's milk, sheep's milk also makes a fine and low-calorie protein cheese. Ricotta can be used in cooked foods, also, where some cheeses, such as mozzarella, can be substituted with great success. Because it is available in whole or skim-milk varieties, you are able to further your focus for lowering fats while retaining all the beneficial nutrients.

Proteins - While we've talked a lot about proteins, you can never say enough about this important fitness base. Many proteins in our diet, however, can get a bit monotonous. Some variances to consider when planning your weekly diet.

Black Beans - These mighty beans are easily prepared and add no carbs. Also high in antioxidants, black beans can give you a bit of substance in a snack, blended for hummus, or in a main course, rolled veggie enchiladas with avocados.

Edamame - Eat them cold, eat them hot, add them to salads or mash them for hummus, edamame has a hard time finding a place where it won't be delicious. Consider the 11 grams of protein per ounce, the added Vitamin C, and fiber gives it more reasons for adding it to your diet plan. Try sauteing them with a bit of olive oil and some herbs for a tasty and nutritious snack, hot or cold.

Greek Style Plain Yogurt - Though this food has been mentioned in more than one chapter, bringing it up again as a protein only adds to its beauty. Staying away from the ones with added toppings and flavors, however, is the only way to really benefit from the doubled proteins over average yogurts without paying a price in added sugars. Put blueberries and toasted oatmeal in the stir, and you have your own nutritious protein without the added waste.

Jerky - With meat proteins offering a somewhat limited preparation choice, add jerky into the mix for great protein and a good alternative for snacks on the go. Choose wisely, as many have added preservatives and fillers. Better yet, dry your own jerky. You can even add veggies into the mix for a little variance.

Quinoa (pronounced *keen'-wah* - at 8 grams per cup, quinoa not only contains a hefty amount of protein, but it also has ample amino acids, to be considered a complete protein. You can add this great source to many of your basic dishes - add to salads and veggie bowls to start the list.

Spreads - Out with the cream cheese, in with the avocado. While the old spreads with maple and pecans or honey and blueberries were delicious, today we know these processed 'cheeses' have little nutrition and tons of sugar. Such is true also with dips - ranch, onion, clam, and queso. But revamping your supplements doesn't have to mean you need to give up the 'extras' you put on carbs and proteins. Take a look at some of the substitutes, in addition to the cheeses you've already read about above.

Avocado - What once was thought to be a soft food full of calories and no benefits, has risen to the king spot of nutri-ent-packed edibles. Avocados do have calories, but the fats are the good ones, and the essential nutrients in just one avocado could put a chicken breast to shame. The fats avocados are so notoriously accused of having, are actually artery-scrubbing, hunger-dulling healthy fats, that can curb appetite cravings too. Along with artery cleansing, plaque which clogs paths to the brain are decreased by these same fats. Look for firm but soft fruit, scoop out the inside, and smash with some other additions if you'd like, such as plain yogurt or lemon juice and herbs. Or just plain, an avocado can definitely stand on its own flavor! This spread goes on just about anything, from toast to tacos. Average 4 grams of protein per fruit.

Nut Butters - Peanuts aren't the only nut you can define as tasty that also can add to your well-rounded fitness plan. A quick pulse or two in a smoothie machine can reduce most nuts down to a spreadable and nutritious food, able to satisfy your need as a quick dip with veggies or fruits, or an addition to oatmeal, breads, and crackers. Think about 2 tablespoons per day, it will give you 7 grams of protein.

Fruit Butters - One really great thing about mashing up a bunch of fruit together is you are able to capture all the nutrients their skins provide, as well as consume it in a different manner, which is good variety for your pallet. You can also mix fruits together, such as peach and plum or blueberry and pear. Throw these in your smoothie blender too, with just a bit of lemon to keep the fruit from turning dark. If you have too much juice, strain it using cheesecloth or a coffee filter, and use it within a day or two, kept in the fridge, or freeze for a cool summer treat. You can also add a bit of cornstarch to the mix if you like a thicker blend to spread.

Whipped Oils with Herbs - Having a whipped oil spread on hand is like having a secret weapon in your nutrition arsenal. Not only can it add beneficial fats to your diet, but the flavor adds a new dimension for your taste buds. Pick an oil you prefer, olive, sunflower, olive, jojoba, or any of the many wonderful choices. Put about ½ cup into your blender with some herbs or flavorings, like basil with a teaspoon of lemon juice, lavender and honey, or oregano. Blend until the oil becomes 'whipped' and thickened (about 3 to 5 minutes), and top this on a sandwich, soup, pizza, or anything else you'd like to give a zip to. Have fun with them!

Greek Style Plain Yogurt - This is a thick, basic spread

which not only doubles the protein intake of typical yogurts - you can add numerous items to it to change it up a bit, including chia seeds, sunflower seeds, poppy seeds, mashed banana, and nut butters. Go to your nutrition counter and see what items you could add to yogurt to make it interesting and new. As you get to know yogurt as a base, you can expand its use to your own likes.

Hummus - Though processed hummus can be a good nutritional food, if you make your own hummus, you'll find more essential nutrients are loaded in it, without all the processed additives and preservatives which will bog down your fitness plan. Canned chickpeas packed in water can also be blended with other foods you like - tomatoes, herbs, peppers (spicy and sweet), avocado, cilantro, sesame seeds, etc. ... You can also mix and match other essential nutrients to make it a powerhouse in your planned fitness diet.

Steroids - This is a case where the 'myth' is a safety issue and popular claims are that steroids are safe to take as supplemental nutrients. Information on steroids is ample, though most of it is written by the manufacturers and sellers of such supplements, favoritizing the use of them as beneficial, particularly in bodybuilding. Research and studies show the use of steroids is detrimental to one's health and can potentially contain illegal substances. Many are listed on the DEA's list of controlled substances and are required to be regulated. Use extreme caution when contemplating taking steroids of any form. Often they are marketed as containing a testosterone 'booster' and are referred to as 'designer steroids' or prohormones, which sidestep the illegality of such ingredients. If labels list these statements or any which sound suspicious, heed the red flag warning and do not add them to your plan. Many of them test positive for anabolic steroids. But aside from this competitive downfall, the risks are high for developing health issues. Stay clear from the glitzy claims and the so-called possible advantages. Unless prescribed by a medical physician, most claims are unproven and could contain illegal substances.

Chapter Summary

• We've been told throughout our lives that some foods are fattening and others are good for you. Recent research and studies have shown us, many of them have been given a false reputation.

• Different preparation styles of the same food can enhance your daily menu, keeping boredom and monotony at bay.

• Many of the foods we used to consume can be updated with nutritious ingredients, making them not only delicious, but advantageous fitness partners.

Now, let's put all this information into action.

CHAPTER TEN: PUTTING THE GAME PLAN IN MOTION

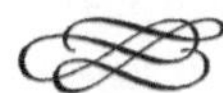

"*With my place on the US Team and the title National won, I felt like I was on top of the world! I was a bit weary, yes, but I wasn't drained. I didn't have weeks of recuperation ahead of me, trying to rebuild the strength I had lost during the competition.*

If I were to go into another challenge soon after this, I would be confident to schedule that challenge, instead of passing it by, thinking I couldn't be at my peak for another demanding event. My body recovered well and could have taken on another competition much sooner than I would have ever guessed.

But I was glad to take the two weeks rest before another 12 weeks of training camp having to do it all over again for the World Championships that August in the UK. Knowing this strategy of supplying different, more digestible and power-boosted foods and supplements while asking the most strenuous of demands, has given me an advantage over my opposition. And that has made all the difference!"

Now that you know how essential nutrients work in your body and how they play key roles in your overall fitness, you can begin to assemble your own, personal, game plan. After all, performance isn't just about weight training!

Choose the goals you want to attain. Do you want to bench press 300 lbs? Do you want to run the Boston Marathon next year? Are you challenging yourself to just get healthier? Choose a goal that you believe you can achieve, but also give yourself a goal that will need some dedicated training to accomplish. Also, keep your time frame in check. Don't begin a plan to bench 300 lbs. by the end of the week when you're pushing 100 lbs. now.

If you are striving for a title, competition, or fundamental change, you may want to consider working with a trainer. He or she can give you the straight talk about your goals and help you become enthusiastic about attaining them. You probably don't need them yelling at you while you're crunching your last 10 sit-ups, but a knowledgeable fitness trainer or nutritionists will set up small goals for you, which will in turn, give you ambition to conquer the next. They will also be able to give you straight talk about supplements and which ones are geared more to your body composition.

Talk about your goals and decide if what you want to achieve is possible in the time limit you may have. At this point, listen to your trainer. They have a keen sense of where you are starting from, and how long it may take to get there. As you already know, the physical body isn't the only thing which has to be considered either. Your dedication, your commitment to follow through, the time it will take, and the consistency which needs to be maintained. All these things, and more, will play into your game plan.

The best part about this time in your fitness planning ... it's exciting, you are working for *you*!

Instead of listening to a trainer and blindly trusting what they say is the truth, you will understand, because you've read this book and can apply all of the things you have learned here. You can intelligently discuss your program and be part of the planning instead of just going through the motions and nodding your head. Perhaps you may come up with a better way to achieve the same results, either with a change to your diet or times of doses. By becoming involved in your program, you will own it and thereby, be more invested and have a better outlook in its success.

Next, by using many of the descriptions and explanations here, decide on the foods you like to eat. What do you enjoy putting in your smoothies? Are carbs important to your overall plan, and if so, which ones would you use in your diet with the least amount of excess?

You know the importance of proteins and how they can make a difference also. Here, you can change it up a bit too, increase your supplemental proteins when doing cardio, and consume meat and fish when you are doing weight training. Mixing it up will give you a variety and keeps boredom at bay. The more you know, the more variety you can use to keep things interesting and delicious while at the same time, giving your body exactly what it needs to achieve your goals.

By knowing which supplements support the essential elements you need in your diet, you have a broader spectrum of choices also. With the variety of foods available, you can prepare these foods in different ways to keep your meals varied while not buying a bunch of different products. Grill your veggies one night and add leftover extras to a rice bowl the next.

Key Strategies to Adopt

-Always have something in the morning before you run, workout, or go to work. Due to the fact your blood sugars are low when you wake, boosting your carb intake will get your system working in a beneficial way. Perhaps a half a bagel or a slice of toast right after you get out of bed. Then, even if you are immediately heading out the door for a run, chances are you've had 20 minutes or so before asking your body to perform, which it will draw for energy from the bagel instead of depleting your muscles.

If you think a slice of toast will cause a major assault on your stomach, start small. Try a small glass of juice, and then move into a solid carb for more substance in a week. Keep in mind, if you add a spread, say cream cheese or butter, it will take extra time for your stomach to digest, making optimum time between eating and beginning your workout longer. Try to forgo the protein until after your workout.

-Make sure you are hydrated. Drink a glass of water before your workout too, so you have available hydration as you move through the exercise. It will also give your ingested carb some extra help to breakdown and be assimilated into your system faster. One ounce of water for every pound of bodyweight is a good, daily guide for needs, maybe ⅛ of this goal is a good start to your day.

-Keep up on your antioxidants to govern free radicals. This is also a good place to consider a supplement dose.

-Make sure you are getting your minerals, as exercise will deplete them. Iron is at the top of the list, especially for women. Include oatmeal, red meats, and spinach into your daily meals, as well as balancing your needs with any supplement you see needed, but don't overdo it. Remember, iron will throw your GI tract off if you consume too much.

-By now, you've realized the benefit of being your own sous chef. Consider taking some time to fix multiple meals and snacks ahead of time, so when you are on the go, it's just a quick grab and you're out the door. By having things ready to go, you'll also be giving yourself an extra advantage to keep to the plan, which gives you results sooner and with more success.

-If you are a woman, don't think this is the time to lose

those 5 stubborn pounds. This isn't the right way to become lean. By depleting your needed nutrients, you won't have the stored carbs available and the risk of muscle breakdown and injury is high without immediate availability.

-In relation to the above statement, make sure you have the carb storage you will need for your competition or event prior to its needed day. The night before, you'll want to top off your resources - if you are overeating carbs, which you know turn to fat, you are doing yourself a disservice, especially when you are striving for a goal and needing the immediate energy. Do not introduce any new idea into your diet plan the day, or even the week before your competition or athletic event. Doing so will throw your system off and it won't have time to adjust to the difference, no matter how beneficial it may promise to be.

-If your competition or workout lasts longer than an hour, plan on refueling during this time. It could be carbs to restore your glycogen reserves or the replenishing of needed electrolyte fluids, the same as you've been taking during your training. Make sure you do both, as they work together to give your system the food for energy as well as the hydration for restoring and enabling absorption of nutrients.

-Always, always, after you finish a competition, workout, or activity, add a protein drink or carb to your restorative routine. You'll have less muscle breakdown and soreness and it will aid tissue and muscle recovery. Electrolytes work well immediately after exercise, teamed with high quality proteins and carbs shortly after, within 30 minutes. Within the hour, try to get a combination of all the essentials in, a whole grain bread sandwich with proteins, lean meat, cheese, or egg work well. Avoid processed carbs, as they delay recovery and could intensify damage you suffered from the workout.

-Six of my favorite foods include

eggs (which contain amino acids, making them a great

choice for muscle building and they transport well when hard-boiled!)

oats (an easily varied and great fuel food to keep energy up, think cooked oatmeal with dried fruits and nuts in a jar for quick snacks)

whey protein (always, and daily in my regime, this is the foundation of my smoothies)

bananas (besides being a handy food, it is an excellent source of potassium and keeps muscles from cramping during workouts and recovery)

peanut butter (great for building muscle tissue, providing great protein amounts and good-for-your heart nutrients)

spinach (beta-carotene and calcium are packed into this versatile food - use in smoothies, omelets, salads, stir-fry, and soups)

-Six of my best recovery foods

chocolate milk (because of the many carbohydrates and proteins, this is a great go-to after workout drink - it assimilates fast in your body and gives you fast recovery)

eggs (enjoy with a meal or vary your intake up by using in a salad or topped on a soup)

greek yogurt (fights muscle inflammation and when coupled with fruit, can give you extra nutrients and antioxidants)

sweet potatoes (replenishes the body with major recovery advantages, adds immunity benefits too, if you strain your muscles or are injured)

avocado (the monounsaturated fat is essential for muscle and joint repair, plus Vitamin B)

water (dehydration can outweigh the benefits of a great workout, so make sure you have plenty of water before, and certainly after, working out, as feeling sick or dizzy doesn't do anyone any good!)

Lastly, if you have read this book thoroughly and abide

by its guidelines, you probably already have or are developing, an intuitive sense of what is good and what is not. By following your instincts and paying attention to your body's signs, each and every step you take to achieving your goal will be an advantage and beneficial in achieving your end result.

CHAPTER SUMMARY

• You now have all the tools and knowledge to assemble a winning fitness diet plan which will support your body's systems and needs, giving you the best possible outcome to achieve your fitness goals.

• By researching the foods you eat, you can easily define the supplements and essential nutrients needed for a balanced eating routine.

• Consuming your supplements in liquid or gel form gives you immediate rewards from the nutrients' bounty.

ADDED ENCOURAGEMENT, GUIDANCE, AND FUN ARE ON the way.

FINAL WORDS AND A FEW TASTY TIDBITS

"Even though I have reached many milestones of which I had no idea how I could accomplish, I am still striving to better myself and my outlook. My consulting and coaching have given me a humble approach to life, while at the same time, it prepares me to be the best Tactical Training Instructor possible.

Being a health & fitness instructor/trainer, I am able to share with others the incredible world of martial arts. By giving to them, especially to the skinny kids who look for confidence and self-worth in an ever-changing world, I believe I can share the precision and strength of martial arts, and teach them, you don't have to be big to be great."

Now you have it, all the information you need to plan, execute, and achieve the best nutritional balance your body has ever known. There is a lot to learn in addition to your supplementing and a well-balanced diet plan - consider workout exercises, agility training, mental preparedness, and so much more.

I commend you for undertaking a diet reboot, I know it isn't an easy task, and many would have been discouraged after the beginning paragraph.

You have done it, you have accomplished a learning challenge which will not only benefit you today, but will remain with you throughout your life. Because you have taken the time to purchase, read, and plan your diet changes with this book, you have proven to yourself you are worthy of a fit body and have the abilities to achieve greatness. Nutrition is a founding block for your fitness program. It is not, however, the only part of a well-nourished and fit body.

Exercise is essential to keep all your systems, circulatory, digestive, nervous, respiratory, cardiovascular, muscular, lymphatic, endocrine, urinary, reproductive, and skeletal, all functioning and working well.

With exercise, you are increasing blood flow, keeping your heart healthy, avoiding stroke, high blood pressure, high cholesterol, and heart disease. You also are keeping diabetes, arthritis, osteoporosis, and aging at bay, by increasing muscle mass and blood circulation.

One of the key reasons many people work out is for the emotional benefits. These highs, or endorphin boosts, are what keep our minds and attitudes feeling good. Endorphins kick in when our bodies would tend to fail, and maintain a positive attitude, even when the exercise is taxing us physically.

Exercise also increases energy levels, especially if you exercise regularly. And the dedication you show when you adhere to an exercise program can carry even the bleakest of days into an accomplished and satisfied attitude.

Weight loss is also a benefit of exercise, and is often, the main motivator for beginning an exercise program. This also contributes to a healthy digestive system and wards off belly fat, which attacks internal organs and can cause many negative attributes including depression, fatigue, and diabetes, to name just a few.

And lastly, but certainly not least, is the soul, the mortar between the bricks. The part of your fitness goals which binds the physical to the mental.

If you approach the well being of your soul, you will be feeding your needs on the inside, where your heart and mind reside. By turning inward to your inner self, you will see how beliefs, self-worth, past accomplishment and defeats, as well as present state of mind, all affect your success in not only your nutrition, but also in your fitness and personal goals.

When you accomplished a task you weren't quite sure you could win, how did you feel?

Exhilarated? Dumb-founded?

Was there a part of you that knew you could do it, or did you have to fight every step of the way, in not only winning physically, but also proving to yourself you could do the task? Healing past wounds, some inflicted by ourselves and others inflicted by outside sources, is one of the key components in any successful achievement. To do this, you need to go within, find the source, mend the wound, and begin the process of building up your confidence to the point of *knowing* you will win this competition. You are capable of greatness. And your achievement goals are only as far away as your ambition to attain them.

Discover the greatness that you are inside. Believe in yourself - do the work on the outside to reach the happiness you can achieve on the inside. It is impossible to have one without the other. When you begin this journey, and begin on any platform you choose (in this case, your successful diet program) you will find gratification and peace in everything you do.

Fitness and health are yours, and with the right tools, you will attain your goals before you know it.

While you contemplate your other options to achieve your ideal self, try some of the recipes I've included below. As you have learned from this book, freshness of the ingredients of your food, and the preparation of your meals are vital keys to making sure your ingredients are exactly what you want and need. They are prepared with the end result in mind - to be very nutritious as well as delicious.

Smoothies - These are a take-me-with-you type of nutrition that is hard to beat. While consuming them directly after making, having one in your hand as you leave your home is always a great idea. Make sure you put your smoothie to go in an insulated cup, as warm fruit tends to discolor and loses its flavor - your smoothie will look like a tan cup of goo with no taste value after a 40-minute commute and a stifled elevator ride to your office.

Strawberry Banana Smoothie - 1 serving

This smoothie can be made any time of the year, but when the strawberries are ripe and available at your grocery store, I'd take advantage of that whenever possible!

- 2 cups fresh or frozen strawberries
- 1 ripe banana
- ½ cup ice cubes
- 1 cup milk or almond milk
- ½ to 1 scoop vanilla whey protein powder

Mix in a blender, pour in large glass, and enjoy.
Some additions or substitutions you may like:

- chia seeds
- 2 tablespoons honey
- greek plain yogurt for milk, for a thicker version

Pineapple Blueberry - 1 serving

This is such a refreshing smoothie. If the banana over-powers the blueberries, using frozen bananas will decrease the intense banana flavor.

- 1 cup fresh or frozen blueberries
- 4 to 5 chunks frozen pineapple, or fresh if you have one cut up
- 1 small or ½ large banana
- 1 cup greek style plain yogurt
- ¾ cups unsweetened almond milk
- 1 scoop vanilla whey protein powder

Mix all ingredients in a blender and blend until desired consistency. You could also add a few nuts to make the texture a bit more bold and interesting. I would use almonds.

Grilled Meats - The only way to have meat, if you ask me, is grilled on a bar-b-q. If this isn't possible, try broiling in your oven on a wired 'grill' in a baking pan. Quick roast red meats with a high temp for oven cooking, around 425 degrees F, for two minutes, and then bake at 325 degrees F to desired doneness. Or, try one of my favorite grilled meat recipes below.

Grilled Chicken Breast

Chicken is a staple as far as training and fitness go. Almost purely all protein with a price tag less than fish, it tops many athletes and nutritionist Top 10 Foods list. But it doesn't take long to grow tired of broiling or roasting chicken, and there's only so much you can do on the grill … or is there?

Here is my favorite recipe for Grilled Chicken Breast, with a couple of variations thrown in to make it interesting.

Basic preparation - Makes 2 Servings

Skin and bone 2 chicken breasts, removing membranes and tendon in the fillet. Place on a grill with medium heat for your preferences, a bit of flavored wood pellets thrown on top for rich smokey tastes. Remove when outside is roasted and the inside is moist and juices run clear (no pink).

Marinated with Lemon Juice and Rosemary

The night before grilling, add chicken breasts to a zip-lock bag with the juice from one lemon and fresh rosemary, removed from the stem and chopped. This marinade can also be used on the chicken while grilling to keep it moist and flavorful – don't baste for the last 2 minutes of grilling.

Almonds Breaded Chicken

Prepare chicken as described above. Before putting on the grill, dip chicken in milk or egg wash and then in slivered almonds. Grill as usual. This crunchy coating adds crunch to your chicken while still keeping the meat tender and flavorful.

Chinese Stir-Fry

The next time you grill chicken, grill twice as much, and save the doubled portions in a storage container in the fridge. Chop up saved chicken into bite-size pieces and stir-fry with vegetables and just a bit of low sodium soy sauce, hoisin, or peanut sauce. Adding a bit of honey to the sauce, or wasabi, will also give it an extra kick. Use whatever vegetables you have on hand, such as onion, zucchini, summer squash, mushrooms, peppers, broccoli, and spinach (quick flash in the pan) for the stir-fry, cook until just tender, and serve over brown rice.

Italian Chicken

Grill chicken as usual. After cooking, serve chicken with nutritious tomato or pizza sauce, or diced tomatoes and a good measure of parmesan. Reheat in the oven and serve with whole wheat pasta.

Crock Pot Chicken

By cooking in the crock pot, the chickens' flavor will not only be enhanced, but the tenderness can't be matched. Put the same skinned, boned, and cleaned chicken breasts as grilling, into a crockpot with vegetables and a can of veggie broth or health-wise soup. Add a bit of water if necessary. Cover and cook throughout the day. You can try this with salsa too, or any canned vegetable you may have from your fall harvest. Chicken can be served over brown rice, whole-wheat pasta, in quesadillas, or fat-free tortillas for tacos. Top with your favorites, and remember to substitute greek style plain yogurt for sour cream.

Use your imagination when grilling chicken. A dry rub shaken in a ziplock bag of your favorite herbs and spices is always a hit, as is basting with a bit of Worcestershire sauce, chili sauce, and balsamic vinegar.

Grilled Salmon Patties with Garlic Habanero Teriyaki Sauce

Salmon patties you have prepared yourself are always the

best. But if you don't have the patience to make them yourself, some frozen patties can be delicious. And you can't beat the ease!

Grill or cook salmon patties to your preference, and top with the following sauce. You can serve a nice side such as greens and citrus salad, which compliments the 'heat' well, and brown rice, or fresh fruit. Your taste buds will wake up after a few bites of salmon, so make sure the side dishes you serve are pleasing and refreshing to counter the sauce.

Garlic Habanero Teriyaki Sauce

This recipe makes 3 cups, so you will have plenty for future meals. Keep in a tightly closed jar in the refrigerator for storing.

- 1 cup soy sauce
- 1 cup grapefruit or orange juice
- ⅓ cup hoisin sauce (low sodium if possible)
- ¼ cup ketchup
- 3 tablespoons white rice vinegar
- ¼ cup golden brown sugar, lightly packed
- 1 habanero pepper, halved and seeded
- 1 tablespoon ground ginger
- 4 cloves fresh garlic, skinned and smashed

Combine all ingredients in a saucepan and bring to a boil. Reduce heat to medium-low and simmer 10 minutes, or until thick, stirring occasionally. Strain sauce and refrigerate leftovers. You may prepare this sauce ahead of time and serve when you have the salmon patties cooked and ready to top.

Pasta - Although some people tend to veer away from pasta, as it is perceived as wasted carbs when trying to lose weight, athletes love the benefits of its preparation and variety in meals. You can top it with sauces, use it in soups, boost an omelet carb intake before an event, or add cold veggies for a portable pasta salad. Below, find one of the most popular recipes in my field, which has its roots in Asia, but a bit of Italian cuisine thrown in for good measure!

Spicy Garlic Butter Linguine - Makes 2 servings

- ½ cup olive oil
- 1 head garlic, cleaned and finely sliced
- 2 cloves garlic, cleaned and finely minced
- 5 ounces dry linguine
- 1 teaspoon dried chili flakes
- 2 tablespoons unsalted butter
- 2 tablespoons soy sauce, low sodium
- 3 tablespoons oyster sauce
- Freshly grated parmesan cheese
- Springs of chopped spring onion (garnish)

Saute the sliced garlic in the olive oil on low heat, being careful to do it slowly, infusing the garlic taste to the oil without browning the garlic. Garlic crisps and burns quickly, so be careful to not let this happen. When it has reached a nice golden color, remove from heat and set it aside. It will continue to cook off the heat.

Cook the linguine according to package directions for al dente. I usually add a bit of olive oil to the water to keep the pasta from sticking together. Drain when cooked.

Heat a medium saucepan over medium-high heat, with 1 tablespoon olive oil and the butter. Add minced garlic and the chili flakes, stirring constantly to marry the flavors. The garlic will soften just a bit, and keep it to a golden color as before.

Add soy sauce, oyster sauce and mix well. Simmer on low for about a minute, then add the cooked pasta, coating the noodles in the sauce, gently stirring and tossing until everything is well combined over low heat. Keep tossing for about one minute while reducing the liquid until it becomes thick and glossy. Serve, topped with cooked garlic slices, parmesan cheese, and spring onion.

~

If you enjoyed this information in this book and it was helpful to you please leave a review.

~

ABOUT THE AUTHOR

George is a devoted full time father, husband and Family Man who places Jesus above all else.   He is a Martial Artist, Martial Arts Instructor with Multiple Black Belts in TaeKwon-Do and Hapkido. He was a TaeKwon-Do National Sparring Champion and a Member of the 2007 USA Team.

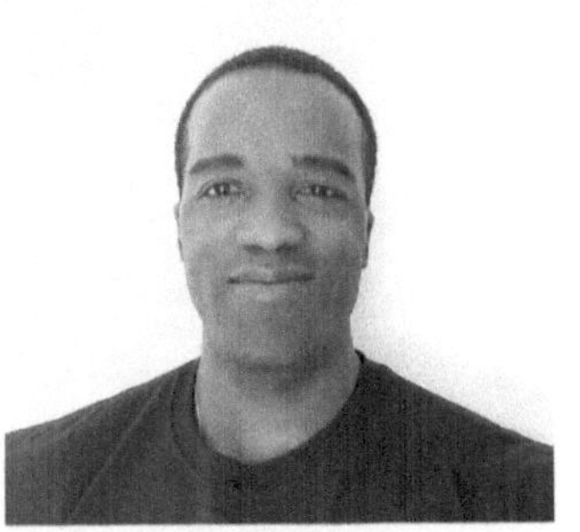

G.E.S. Boley Jr.

He is a Defensive Tactical Training Instructor, with training in hand to hand combat, stick and knife fighting and Freestyle Grappling. He is a health and fitness instructor and trainer, certified sports nutritionist, business entrepreneur, real estate investor, property manager, business consultant and coach.

Along with training certifications George has a Bachelor's degree in Marketing and an MBA in Business. George has many life experiences and is passionate about learning and helping people in need.

He is a Certified International Instructor with the ITF, Certified Fitness Trainer and Certified Sports Nutritionist.

SPECIAL BONUS!

Get this additional Supplements that Help with Obesity and Fat Guide 100% FREE!

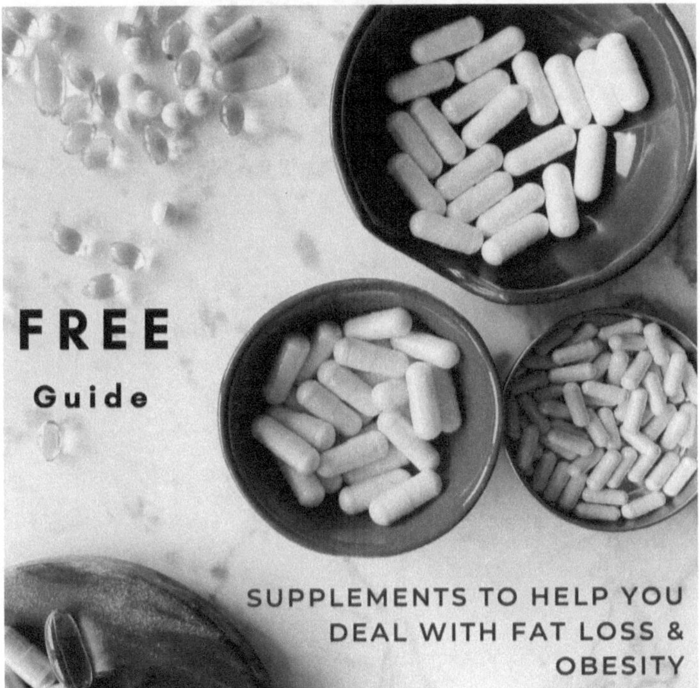

Many others are currently enjoying the benefits of insider access and the ability to get my books for FREE!

Yes, 100% FREE!

If you want insider access plus this <u>Supplements that Help with Obesity and Fat Guide</u>, all you have to do is **click the qr code below** to claim your offer!

REFERENCES

Active.Powering the world's events and activities.retrieved June 2020 at https://www.active.com/

CHAMP Uniformed Services University.Human Resources Performance Resources.Total force systems.retrieved June 2020 at https://www.opss.org/

Cleveland Clinic Healthline.Feature health topics.retrieved June 2020 at https://www.healthline.com/

Harvard Health Publishing Harvard Medical School.Trusted advice for a healthier life.retrieved June 2020 at https://www.health.harvard.edu/

Harvard T.H. Chan School of Public Health.The nutrition source.retrieved June 2020 at https://www.hsph.harvard.edu/

MaxLiving.Health and fitness leaders.retrieved June 2020 at https://maxliving.com/

MedicineNet. Drugs and supplements. retrieved June 2020 at https://www.medicinenet.com/script/main/hp.asp

Shape. Fitness. Healthy eating. retrieved June 2020 at https://www.shape.com/

The Healthy. Newsletter. retrieved June 2020 at https://www.thehealthy.com/

Uniformed Services University. The department of defence dietary supplement resource. Consortium for health and military performance. Operation supplement safety. retrieved June 2020 at https://www.opss.org/

Wikipedia. Reference definitions. retrieved June 2020 at https://www.wikipedia.org/

www.ingramcontent.com/pod-product-compliance
Lightning Source LLC
Chambersburg PA
CBHW031239250726
48655CB00005B/2024